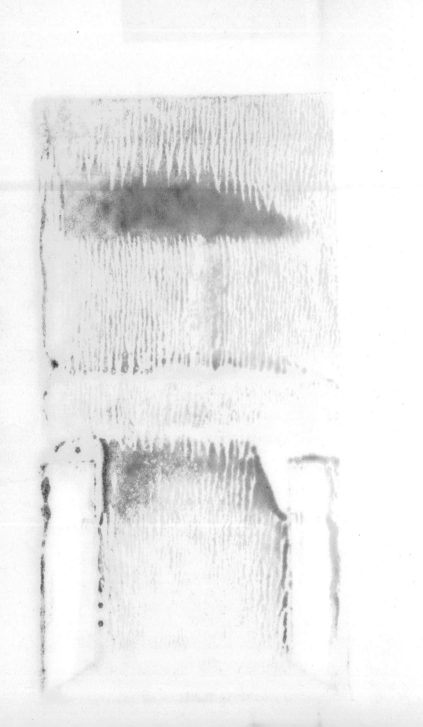

Also by Lois Wheeler Snow

China On Stage

A Death with Dignity

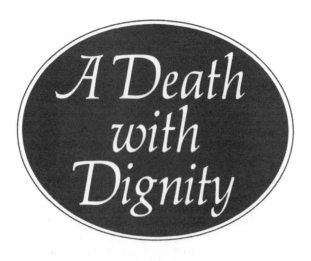

A Death with Dignity

WHEN THE CHINESE CAME

Lois Wheeler Snow

Random House   New York

Copyright © 1974, 1975 by Random House, Inc.

All rights reserved under International and Pan-American
Copyright Conventions. Published in the United States by
Random House, Inc., New York, and simultaneously in Canada
by Random House of Canada Limited, Toronto.

Library of Congress Cataloging in Publication Data
Snow, Lois Wheeler.
A Death with Dignity.
1. Cancer—Personal narratives. 2. Snow, Edgar,
1905–1972. 3. Medicine, Chinese. I. Title.
RC263.S62S58   362.1'9'699400924   [B]   74–26640
ISBN 0–394–49673–6

"The Burial of Edgar Snow"
originally appeared in somewhat different form in
The New Republic.

Grateful acknowledgment is made to Dr. Joseph Needham
and *China Now* to reprint an excerpt from a speech
by Dr. Needham which appeared in this journal of
The Society for Anglo-Chinese Understanding. Also
to *Eastern Horizon Magazine* for permission to
reprint and excerpt from " In a Chinese Hospital"
by E. M. Christiansen (Vol. XII, No. I, 1973).

Design by Bernard Klein

Manufactured in the United States of America

9 8 7 6 5 4 3 2

To
Jean and Mary and Trudie

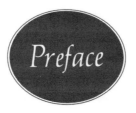

Preface

Death lingered in our home; we were busy and didn't notice. Death gazed from my husband's eyes; I thought, "He's tired, he needs a rest." Cancer crept into body tissues; Ed frowned. "I have a headache," he sighed, "I'll lie down a bit."

Pale sun pecked at shriveled garden stalks, icicles dripped off the courtyard roof tiles. Our typewriters danced; reworked papers heaped high. We paused for rest —midmorning coffee, drinks before dinner, a walk through winter-rye-green fields in sight of Mont Blanc's frozen peak across the gray Geneva lake. Unsuspected, unseen, death waited—tucked into time.

A Death with Dignity

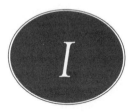

It was March 1971 when Ed and I, back from a trip to China, returned to our home in Switzerland, a few weeks before China woke up a war-weary world with the sprightly bounce of ping-pong balls. In 1970, the year before the People's Republic entered the United Nations, Ed, on another visit there (the only of his many trips on which I was his companion), had again acquired enough facts, figures, photos, interviews and insight to satisfy the most exigent investigator. On return to the shelter of our adopted Swiss home, we worked over these together, day after day —China, for that time, *our* world. It permeated our talk and piled up, neatly labeled, in slides and films on dining-room chairs and the long rosewood table Ed had brought from Peking a decade before. We had it crammed into diaries and scribbled in notebooks, we tailored it into manuscripts and magazine articles and, with the bulky information, formed outlines, paragraphs, and chapters of our books. We felt full and alone, sharing our knowledge, immersed in work.

Death came two months and a day after an operation performed for carcinoma of the pancreas, not quite a year after Ed's return from China. Relief following major surgery had turned quickly to renewed suffering; Ed termed it "postoperative," canceled a planned return to the East, and put his diminishing strength into finishing the book he was writing about the Cultural Revolution. He died before it was completed.

No one could have saved his life. The skillfulness of surgeons and doctors in attendance, his own basic good health and determination to live, proved vanquishable by disease undetected in that strong body for perhaps two years. A "miracle" was not to be. Mankind has had other things to do than find the causes or cures for cancer.

I had sought help throughout the world. It came from many places and in many forms; we were grateful for all. My attempt to tell of this crisis is not because it happened to my husband under unusual circumstances, but because what occurred is, I believe, of relevance to others who, when sickness intrudes and dying defies both the bonds of love and the medical apparatus that has up to then been protection, insurance, guarantee, do not know where else to turn, or what is wrong, or why. Special though we were—for we belong to that minority who have ready access to civilization's privileges—we were unable to cope with the problems that confronted us in the midst of modern scientific techniques and the generously offered resources many friends placed at our disposal. I believe I would not have understood the *why,* the reasons for our dilemma, if a medical team from the People's Republic of China had not arrived to change the pattern of care and to ease the encroachments of even terminal illness by helping family, professionals, and the patient himself participate in preventing humiliation in the face of death. The difference was not in more or better Chinese technical knowledge in the treatment of cancer—the world shares what breakthroughs have been made so far—but in an attitude toward the illness, the patient, and all engaged in the struggle of one person against relentless disease. Everyone in touch with our home was affected by these men and women who had traveled so far to apply the principles of behavior that form their daily lives. It was a profound experience in sharing, one that sometimes occurs between close friends, sometimes between strangers in an emergency, but not often in our society between patient, relatives, friends, and a group of doctors and nurses unhampered and unstinting in their efforts of care.

I find it fitting that this gift of direct, focused concern came from the country my husband had spent a lifetime trying to explain to a too-often hostile world. Perhaps the miracle we so longed for was simply in these people and the life they lead, which allows them the spirit and space to behave with a fuller sense of what humanity means. I know from my own time there, and from others who have participated in or witnessed the developments there,* that the attitude I speak of is inherent in the ideology of new

* For example: *Serve the People*, by Victor and Ruth Sidel; *Away With All Pests*, by Joshua S. Horn; *Women and Child Care in China*, by Ruth Sidel; "The Physician and the Quality of Life," by E. Grey Dimond, in the *Journal of the American Medical Association*, Vol. 228, No. 9 (May 27, 1974).

China and that through this the character of medical service has changed. Before he himself benefited from it, Edgar Snow had written about medical practice in the People's Republic as "a radical change which has significance for the poverty-stricken disease-ridden people of Asia, Africa and Latin-America, and indeed for people everywhere . . . The new health policy in China will have repercussions throughout the world." *

If our hospital personnel, our medical teaching schools, the members of our medical professions, can incorporate into our so different society this concept of total effort which embraces the patient and the patient's family—an ideal demonstrated by the Chinese in our home—then we shall be further ahead in the treatment of our ill and dying. An essential part of that ideal lies in changes that would humanize the ever-increasing mechanical conditions of our present-day medical care. These can come about through the response of citizens—social workers, paraprofessionals, nonprofessionals—to the demand for immediate, tangible help for all sick people, not for charity's sake but for the sake of all, rich and poor, who in falling ill in our society, and dependent on our incomplete health services, risk loneliness, neglect and additional unnecessary pain.

It was not because of any technical medical superiority or undisclosed scientific knowledge that the presence of the Chinese counted so enormously. It was mainly because of an attitude. It is responsibility for one's own behavior within the communal group, and beyond, with political-

* *The Long Revolution* (New York: Random House, 1972; Vintage Books paperback edition, 1973).

6

ideological consciousness cementing the relationships between people. It is attention paid to others with self-examination as a principle; it is a striving, a "struggle" (their term) to become that "new man," that ideal set up by China through the conscious practice of Mao Tse-tung political philosophy. I cannot say it is totally accepted in China today, nor that it has been fully achieved (there would not have been a Cultural Revolution, and other revolutions forecast for the future, if that were true), but it *is* widespread and it *is* impressive, particularly to someone coming from our competitively motivated, self-protected, self-concerned society. That our case was particular, that the situation (in a personal as well as in a larger sense) was special, is not to be denied. But the fundamental motivation that led the medical team to our home from China is felt throughout that country. Perhaps it is most dramatically apparent in the field of medicine, where the former rigidity of medical practice has been broken, as well as new ground gained in the application of preventive methods and care of the sick, in joint action between the people and what used to be in old China the elite medical personnel concentrated in the cities and treating mostly the privileged well-to-do.

This medical revolution stems from a commitment to "serve the people," engendered by a society that not only equates relationship with obligation in communal purposefulness involving each individual with the whole, in a struggle to transform life there for the betterment of all, but equally important, provides the social structure and doctrines that allow and encourage, if not demand, that this commitment be carried out. It has nothing to do with prestige or power, nor with monetary motivation or ability to pay. It is a principle of service instilled in the Chinese from the beginning of life, through political education rooted in their socialist ideology.

The why of this is in China's history; its development and continuation is in China's future, linked with the rest of the world's in interdependent and precarious balance. Its application is in China's present. The essence was seen in our home when the Chinese came, and it is through this experience that I can best make it clear. It is a simple story, but in it may be a future that will affect us all.

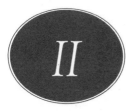

II

When my husband fell gravely ill, the Chinese government responded as to a special friend. Why it did lies in a history that forged durable bonds between Chinese Communist revolutionaries and a non-Communist American who all his life supported in his own country the democratic form of government brought about by his own countrymen's revolution long before that of the Chinese, and who wrote in 1962, in the introduction to his last complete book on China:

> The area of freedom of inquiry . . . [is] of wholly negative value if used only to serve narrow interests of private ownership while censoring the general interest of the public enlightenment and welfare; and a freedom which will soon lose all meaning if those who possess it, on the American side of the frontier, do not more energetically use it to reveal the truth about ourselves as well as the black, the white and the gray about people and systems on the other side.

> The greatest danger which has all along faced America, as Walter Lippmann has eloquently observed, is not communism, but whether we can "to ourselves be true," and whether we can "find our strength by developing and applying our principles, not in abandoning them." *

This need to know (he *was* from Missouri) led him to explore and explain the historic necessity of the Chinese revolution and gained him the confidence of the makers of that revolution, and it was the universal concept and ideological creed of the Chinese Communists that allowed them the openness and largeness of mind to respond with unlimited help to a stricken foreigner outside the boundaries of their country. When Edgar Snow met Mao Tsetung again, in 1960, eleven years after China's liberation, the Chairman said to him, "I haven't changed and you haven't changed." The friendship was based on the probity of two human beings who understood each other's different worlds.

Of course it would be as rare in China to place four doctors and several nurses in a private home as it would be in any other country. The kind of care, the attitude of the people caring, is what is of relevance to those outside the unusual circumstances of our case. If the experience had not been so intimately mine, or even if it had been and I had not had the background to understand its dimensions, I might have accepted it with profound gratefulness, as a favor granted us only, without applicability to others. I knew this was not true. I had been to China.

Our trip there, in 1970–1971, had been special, too—

* *Red China Today: The Other Side of the River,* by Edgar Snow. Revised and updated edition. (Random House, 1971; Vintage Books, 1971).

we were the first Americans to be invited to visit as the country was opening up after the tumult of the Cultural Revolution—and it foreshadowed the coming change of relations between China and the United States. I became a participant in that event, on an October day when nearly a million people packed Peking's Tien An Men, the Gate of Heavenly Peace, in celebration of the twenty-first anniversary of the People's Republic. An avenue-wide parade of marching students, tumbling Peking opera acrobats, peasants spinning in folk dance, ballerinas seemingly frozen in arabesques, and costumed workers astride gigantic floats, khaki-green soldiers swirling red banners, national minority groups in billows of Korean silk and embroidered jackets from Tibet poured steadily past the awesome arches beyond the moat, past the erect figure at the exact center of the ancient gate—Mao Tse-tung.

I stood beside my husband on the west end of the balcony down the line of guests invited to view the panorama from that towering height, conscious that the holiday-gay red and white signboard across the far side of the huge square bore strident words: "Peoples of the world, unite to defeat the U.S. aggressors and all their running dogs." We felt a tug at our backs; the familiar face of Chou En-lai focused into view.

"Come," he said pleasantly, "someone wants to see you."

A blur of spectators limited vision as the Premier escorted us through rows of people into the presence of a Mao Tse-tung taller than I had imagined, thinner than pictures indicated, steady-eyed and grave. Caught in the click of cameras, the moment became a tiny eternity as the Chairman took my hand and I sought in his older face the young man of Anyuan, Chingkangshan, the Long March, Yenan. *"Ni hao,"* we said to each other and moved to the marble balustrade, Ed and I taking a place on either side of Mao Tse-tung in full view of the multitude below. As at the far end of a kaleidoscope, the pageant proceeded, my hand resting on the railing next to the hand of the leader of China; moving my eyes sideways, I could see his famous mole. It was a speck of history in the making—two lone Americans symbolizing an eventful change.

Back in the intimacy of our Peking Hotel room, sipping hot green tea, I asked why *that* had happened—we *Americans* in front of China's millions, side by side the Chairman. Ed nodded and reminded me that the Chinese never do anything publicly without a reason. Subsequently that picture of Ed and the Chairman was featured in Chinese news services and picked up by the world press. (I got cut out in most publications but comforted myself that, after all, I *had* been there.)

Later, traveling west, we saw the Chinese countryside changed beyond the dreams of yesterday's beggar peasants: Sian, where Chiang Kai-shek, tumbling from might to capture in nightdress, had faced the inevitability of compromise; Yenan, cradle city of Chinese Communists; Pao-an, refuge of revolutionaries terminating the Long March in the loess country layered by dust blown down from the Gobi Desert centuries ago. We sped in modern trains across the wheat fields of the Northeast where we toured the great steel plant at Anshan (the first time I ever took the opportunity to look at blast furnaces) and gaped at the cabbage-draped balconies above the streets of Shenyang, prepared for coming winter calm. Peasants opened homes in commune brigade villages to share meals of autumn abundance with us: squash, millet, melons, red tomatoes and golden pears, chicken, pork, steaming noodles and the bright, soft persimmons that leave no pucker in the mouth.

China's worn beauty unfolded as we covered the miles —stretches of dusky land dotted by thatched roofs reminiscent of the northern French countryside, where similar wisps of smoke head up to lonely skies; earthen villages where unpaved streets bore the tracks of newly acquired tractors, and small bookstores meant peasants had something to read on winter evenings. Not only that—it meant they *could read*. The sense of change was deepened for me by Ed, who had known the country from the infancy of its revolution and through the subsequent years after the founding of the People's Republic in 1949.

I was afterward to see, in a different sweep of travel, an even wider view of this metamorphosis—later, when Ed was no longer there as my companion and I returned to China to ride and walk beside his friends, now become mine, in Szechuan, Hunan, Hupei, Kiangsi, seeking the people to extend thanks for the care brought by them to our home in Switzerland.

But there, at that time, was Ed. Together we slept on country kangs (the traditional toast-warm mud-brick beds of peasant origin), climbed over coal mines brought into existence by the local people's determination, boated on reservoirs of deep blue where water had been precious as life before, feasted on fresh fish in formerly arid villages, rested in orchards under trees planted in earth-filled holes man-made out of solid rock. Ed pointed out the differences. Many of these places he had known at another time, when it had not been uncommon to see women with breasts shriveled to dangling leather thongs and babies dying from lack of mother's milk. He had witnessed the periodic and catastrophic famines of the past, the filth and rats, the gangsters and painted ladies, the child slaves and the neck-shackled conscripts. He knew the young and the aged beggars, the wasted coolies, the ravage of opium and war, the desolate, eroded soil. I had learned all this from him; the knowledge of that past deepened the sight of the present.

Driving over the Shensi mountain roads, Ed drew my attention to the terraced slopes, where formerly a worm-eaten pear had been a prize to share with hungry companions. Shopping for mementos and gifts in far-flung department stores, we mingled with the healthy citizens of China who could at last afford an extra padded jacket, a pretty blouse, a mechanical toy for the kids, a strong bike, a radio set or some model Peking opera records. Like Mr. and Mrs. Pied Piper, we were followed through city streets by streams of children, play-dirty or bath-clean, wide-eyed, open-mouthed, grinning, or shy at the sight of Western foreigners, but healthy and well-fed as never before, these offspring of poor peasants and workers.

Students cooperated in explaining the upheaval of education during the Cultural Revolution; actors, and dancers in toe slippers scratched from performances on threshing grounds or factory floors, told us about the new content in the theatre. Young barefoot doctors, men and women, demonstrated the acupuncture technique taught to them by People's Liberation Army medics in tiny, tidy country-side clinics they themselves had built, and young guides showed us China's agricultural and industrial products in the huge display halls of Canton's Trade Fair building. The change in the activities and status of "Ms. China" paled some Western efforts at Women's Liberation in depth and scope, bringing legal equal rights and participation that had dramatically improved the position of the female half of China. This drastic change—to be considered a contributor to the future, to have the choice of marriage, of bearing children, to be able to feed and care for them—meant health, security, dignity and assurance for countless women. Formerly, proliferation had been the way of protecting a family against the high rate of infant mortality, to guarantee a sufficient number of *sons* to ensure support in old age: in Peking I met a peasant woman whose name, Wang San-to, translates into "Three Too Many." Her sister's name is "Four Too Many."

At times we experienced frustration, for in their eagerness to have us understand—inspire us with—this second revolution, the Chinese sometimes presented us with models, while we wanted to see the different problems they were still having with their Cultural Revolution. All was not perfect, and Ed was eagle-eyed and thorough—that was his training. He didn't take to bureaucratic mentality in any form, pre– or post–Cultural Revolution.

I was fascinated. Soaking up the centuries, I filled notebook after notebook. My diary reads: "China with all its richness, still poor. China with all its newness, still old—despite great economic progress and industrial development, a country only beginning to realize its huge potential, a country where seemingly nothing is intentionally wasted—neither people nor talent, where changes in motivation are producing a responsible and responsive citizenship in a country that was second to none in corruption and greed."

Seeing brought home the differences between life and death, decency and indecency, neglect and security: the absence of hungry and homeless; the termination of epidemics, of oppressive taxation, of destitution; the enormous lessening of crime; the freedom from drugs; the national medical care available to everyone; and the national education that had almost done away with illiteracy in less than two dozen years. Impressive as all this was—this physical benefit—more impressive to me was the *spirit* of the Chinese people, through a social system which instills and implements a consciousness of service that motivates and mobilizes its young and old: lively, buoyant, dignified, demonstrated by the closeness of family life without protective selfishness, the integration between children and adults, the open respect and responsibility for others, the greatly reduced concentration on I—*me*. A particularly striking aspect was the intense political participation and involvement of individuals in a collective learning process that forms the people of China into an energetic, attentive, functioning *citizenship*.

In five months' time our diaries became chock-a-block full; we both wrote books about our stay.* It was pre–ping-pong; the word "acupuncture" had not yet gained its careless inclusion in the vocabulary of the West.† After we

* *The Long Revolution*, by Edgar Snow (*op. cit.*). *China On Stage*, by Lois Wheeler Snow (Random House, 1972; Vintage Books, 1972).

† Dr. Samuel Rosen calls the often unscientific application, here in the United States, of China's valid acupuncture, "quackupuncture." (*New*

returned to our portion of the universe, some people believed us and some did not. Now that China is no longer an "anathema," more people accept what Ed had been writing about for years. Other Americans are now going to, and writing about, the People's Republic, no longer cut off by their government from one fifth of the world. For two decades, space had been sparse in the United States for objective accounts of China's hard-won achievements. The blight of McCarthyism had spread across the United States, and Edgar Snow's reportage did not conform to its demands. During that time, in lieu of dealing with contemporary proceedings, he wrote an autobiography (published), several stories for his children (unpublished), and completed the transformation of the little barn behind our house into the studio he had long desired—wondering when he'd appear in print again. That event seemed even further away after he put up his carpentry tools; it wasn't long before we advertised the studio as an apartment and rented it to a young couple who had a regular income.

A journalistic career, begun in 1929 in the newspaper world of Shanghai, had taken this American from the Middle West into the heart of Asia's struggle; he knew what he saw and he had seen more of what made up modern China than any other American journalist over a period of forty-four years. When he arrived there, at the age of twenty-three, he had been "every youth, full of curiosity and wide open to the world." * In 1937, seven

---

York Times, May 28, 1974.) Dr. E. Grey Dimond: "How Can I Get a Visa to China?"

* *Journey to the Beginning* (Random House, 1958; Vintage Books, 1972).

years after a first assignment in the Far East, his startling account of the Chinese Communists and their revolution appeared under the title *Red Star Over China*.* The book, eventually a world classic, brought him fame and respect from some quarters, and scorn and suspicion from others. *Red China Today: The Other Side of the River*, based on his prolonged stay in China in 1960, brought him the same. He carried all with balance and a sense of humor. (A friend with similar qualities recently remarked "Ed had lovely friends and lousy enemies.")

Ed saw only the commencement of international change toward China, enough to make him want to remain longer on this "dear, cruel, indifferent and wonderful Earth," as he wrote in a note, in spite of the battle it meant to continue living. A less vigorous person might have claimed the illness, succumbed on the operating table, submitted to defeat. Though it was hell to watch, I shared and supported his fight.

Death occurred at the very moment his life work became justified, bringing posthumous recognition from many who had ignored, or jeered, in the past. He left eleven books behind, a coverage of contemporary history not on China alone, some of which had been reviewed in the nation's press under such headings as "Snow Job." He was neither rich nor received, except in and by those who appreciated the perception of his reporting and the breadth of his observation. His son and daughter, and I, have gained from him far more than earthly goods.

* First published by Random House in 1938; revised edition published by Grove Press in 1968, and in an Evergreen Books paperbook edition in 1973.

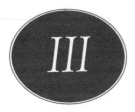

III

From the moment I met Ed my life was wrapped in his, and China became a center. My career in New York's theatre continued after our marriage—I love acting and if I hadn't met Ed, I probably would now be a middle-aged character actress bumping about on tour—but my world enlarged through his. Theatre had meant such a complete world to me that in spite of some political participation (my novice speech, in support of a maverick congressman, had been off the back of a truck on a New York City streetcorner; while enthusiastic, I was scared stiff and must have been pretty unintelligible), I remained fairly innocent of the scope and causes of world social problems. On the other hand I felt that Ed, absent from the States through participation in tumultuous revolution and World War II, was somewhat apart from the realities of *my* world. After reading the script of what I considered a prestigious Broadway production in which I had been offered a part, he asked, sincerely puzzled, "Why do you want to do *that*?" I briskly commented on how far *he* was from the scene. Undismayed, he sent me a dozen red roses on opening night—and the play won the Drama Critics Award for the year. Together with him I began to develop as the partner of a thinking, involved human being who loved life and sought truth, and later as the mother of two new human beings who were going to grow up in the world we had helped create. When our son, Christopher, was not a year old, the Korean War began. We heard the report over the car radio while searching for a picnic spot in Connecticut. I looked at our baby—and at Ed. What would the world be like in another twenty years? The thought was enough to make a mother grow up several notches.

But even before Chris was born, my horizons had expanded. I traveled a lot with Ed, in and out of the United States. In Mexico for the first time, I writhed at the gulf between extremely rich and extremely poor. "Why doesn't it bother *you*?" I asked Ed accusingly. He answered by verbal pictures of India and China, whose poverty paled that of Mexico's, singeing the eyes wherever one turned. It was knowledge knit into his experience, but to be worked against—not shouted about.

In 1947 we drove, in an ancient Renault *"quatre chevaux,"* through France and Italy and England, countries bearing the devastation of recent war like beggars' rags. Only Switzerland stood out pristine, stable and whole. I remember that first morning when after driving across dirty, bedraggled France, we crossed the frontier, found a picture-postcard hotel and breakfasted on real café au lait, croissants, fresh butter and jam. Ed, watching me lick the last crumbs off my fingers, ordered us both a big dish of ice cream. Afterward we lived for a while in a high-ceilinged Bernois apartment perched over the medieval city's river, and I boned up on high school shorthand to take notes during the news interviews Ed handled with ease and depth. He was good, and hard, at work.

Back at home we lived in uptown and downtown New York, and once in Hollywood, where I made a "major" picture and Ed wrote. When we "settled down" after the birth of our son, we chose Sneden's Landing on the Hudson River above the George Washington Bridge. We had been married there on a May day in 1949 in the company of a few close friends, including Ed's brother Howard, and Agnes Smedley, whose books on China were important contributions to my knowledge of that country.* There we made other friends and there Ed carried on the river love he had borne from childhood on the shores of the Missouri. I remember our kitchen crawling with live crabs brought back in buckets from an outing with Sam Zimbalist, who entertained us with his violin during the cooking—Ed the chef. (I couldn't bear plunging crabs into boiling water, but I could eat them with relish once they were cooked.) There Agnes, who shared Ed's culinary enthusiasm (if not his originality—his "recipe" for "tree ear omelet" included dubious fungi gathered from forest barks), topped off her specialties of Oriental pilaf and apple pie by singing "On Top of Old Smokey" and dancing the Chinese *yang-ke*

---

* *Battle Hymn of China* (New York: Alfred A. Knopf, 1943); *The Great Road: The Life and Times of Chu Teh* (New York: Monthly Review Press, 1946).

while telling tales of her days in Yenan—and it was from Sneden's that she, covered by a rug in the back seat of a car, was spirited out from under FBI surveillance. Publicly humiliated, prevented from going to China by a U.S. passport limited to England, she died in London after an operation on a stomach ulcer and, perhaps, a broken heart. Her love for China was immense and a lot of it affected me—as did the fact that she was hounded to death because of it.

There were, too, walks amid the dogwood trees high above the Palisades, drives and sails along the river—and Ed took delight in crossing to the other shore by ferryboat, just for fun. It was easy for me to commute to the theatre in Manhattan across the bridge, and it was tranquil in the countryside where Ed preferred to write.

Later we moved across the state line to New Jersey, a step away, and there, in the outsized Georgian-columned house we bought, we felt we'd live the rest of our lives. It was one of many houses to follow, but we didn't know that then. In spite of subsequent residences we continued for years to call that corner of the globe "home."

They were happy days, a mixture of theatre and literary worlds, of child raising and processions of animals— rabbits, kittens, dogs, the two sheep Ed brought back one day in lieu of the lawn mower he'd gone out to buy (they cropped everything except the lawn), of visiting actors, journalists, scientists, poets and peasants, and eventually of blacklisted and blacklisters. Calls from twin-clad FBI agents became frequent; Ed wryly advised them to read his books instead of asking uninformed questions. He believed in information but not in informing, as some others did. Faces flash out from the past. Some are gone and some remain;

some are sullied and some shine true. It made a difference at the time—it still does—but Joseph McCarthy is dead and we now face even graver problems.

I would have loved to go to China long before I did. In 1951, soon after our daughter, Sian, was born, Ed received an invitation from the People's Republic of China to spend a year there, to investigate, to interview, to write. The children and I were included. I dropped the television script I was memorizing from one hand and the scrambled eggs I was stirring with the other. "Let's go!" I said. Ed said no. We obviously couldn't afford to pay our own way, no publication in the United States would or could send us, and we couldn't go as guests of China—no one in the country would accept Ed's reports if the Chinese government paid our expenses. I understood. I swept up the eggs and resigned myself to unemployment insurance to keep up our credit at a local grocery store. Though I was nearing a year's run on Broadway, the money that made the difference for us was from the increasingly rare television parts that came my way.

I didn't realize I had been blacklisted on all but a few programs (I did keep a running part on a soap opera) until told so by a television director who suggested I do something about it. I did—and found that the dossier against me included a hodgepodge of petitions I had signed against capital punishment and Southern lynchings, some organizations I had never belonged to, and some overstated credits I had given myself when seeking a job without enough experience to get me into an agent's office. At the end of my half-hour interview with the network "vice-president in charge of blacklisting" (*my* term), he pierced me with cold eyes and asked if I had ever been to Brooklyn. I acknowledged that I had gone to Brooklyn Heights several times to visit friends. That noted, he asked me more coldly for my *real* name.

"As stated," I replied, surprised. "I have no other."

"Are you not Miriam Oppenheimer?" he shot at me.

I blanched. That was it? An alias? I invited the man to the Cort Theatre any time he wished to see me in the role I had played for hundreds of performances—that of the young refugee from a Nazi-occupied country who, escaping the concentration camp that devoured her parents, had gone to an aunt's home in Brooklyn: the part I played was "Miriam Oppenheimer." So much for the FBI. The vice-president seemed abashed, but I never got another job on that network.

It didn't help later when James Reston included Ed's name in a "mixed bag of Communists and liberals" on the front page of the *New York Times*. After our lawyer got in touch with him, Mr. Reston called Ed and apologized but nobody else heard his remarks, except possibly the people who were tapping our phone. The *Times* printed Ed's letter of protest and Reston's rather roundabout reply in the Letters to the Editor section, but a good deal of damage had been done. It was a bad blow in a bad time and I couldn't help but admire Ed's objectivity—he continued his respect for both Mr. Reston and the *New York Times*. Eventually I found myself not only blacklisted on television but witch-hunted on my campaign for election to the Board of Education in our small New Jersey town. There had been other fuel for the latter fire: at one of the children's birthday parties we had hung a pair of Japanese paper fish out on the porch to welcome our children's small guests. Word quickly got around that the Snows had Chinese Communist symbols flying in front of their house. We never really lived that down in New Jersey, and what with that and similar offenses I lost the election, albeit by a narrow margin.

It has been said that we left the United States because of such blacklisting and harassment. Actually we drifted away in a physical sense almost by accident, seeking to earn the living, and the freedom to work, that had been curtailed at home during that period of political irresponsibility. Ed had watched grasping men become powerful in the native country he loved and he had watched people overcome grasping men in the country he also loved—China. Because his books and articles dealt factually with both countries, his earning capacity was severely affected. He eventually accepted a job that came out of the blue of Ohio. He wanted it—and not only to pay bills. A position as a teacher with the International School of America, an airborne classroom whose year's trip around the world offers students a chance to live in many countries as they study, gave Ed the opportunity to reacquaint himself with the East. He joined for the school year 1959–1960 and I jumped at the offer to live in a friend's house in Switzerland during the interim. We planned a year abroad; we stayed on, as U.S. citizens, making new friends and retaining old ones, while educating our children in the calm of the little country that became a second home. It was less expensive than the United States, clean, quiet and beautiful. Ed found it possible to publish in the European press, to earn a living again, to return to China to pick up the métier cut short by the bullying of McCarthyites and those cold warriors who specialized in screaming "Red."

U.S. passport restrictions extended to more countries at that time than now, and in Washington, China was *the* villain. Ed, with a visa in his pocket (the Chinese had declined to insert it in a passport that bore the words "Not valid for travel to Communist China"), got financial backing from *Look* magazine and was therefore able to legally circumvent the travel ban; the State Department refused my request to accompany him and behind I stayed, unable to make two trips East with him in the sixties. (When Ed arrived without me, the Chinese said, "Where's your wife?" It seemed odd to them that Americans could believe that husbands were separated from wives in the People's Republic while it was the United States that had prevented me from accompanying my husband to China.)

It was not until our visit in 1970 that I could begin work in common with this husband of some twenty years, as we refocused on each other after our son and daughter had become adults and we a "couple" once again. The two of us found a different cooperation, a culmination of experience, blended, sure. China had much to do with this because China is a new experience that sparks new thoughts and that in itself makes one fresh again.

When we kissed each other good-bye at the airport in Peking at the end of December in that year of 1970, I was joyous and replete. Ed would join me in California after a few more weeks in China; I was eager to see my childhood home—I was born and raised in the San Joaquin Valley, and my roots lie buried in its warmth.

Sparkling waves of the Pacific Ocean lapped at San Francisco's shores; the plane seemed suspended in sunshine over the city where my California family waited to greet me. There was a dreamlike unreality in plunging from China to the United States in the time span of jet propulsion. A night's stopover in Hongkong had not been enough to bridge the physical and ideological separation. I had a feeling of uniqueness; there were few who understood. When a minx of a child, age six or so, seated by a window facing the Peninsula's expanse of water, asked me "Where *is* China?" I pointed out the mauve tips of the Golden Gate barely visible through the sun-touched fog. "If you could stand on that bridge and look straight out across the ocean, if you could look all the way across to the other side, you'd see China." Not being a geographer, she looked hard out the window. "I wish I could see it," she sighed. I wished she could too. I had, and part of me had stayed there.

Pre-Chrismas Califorina was a supermarket of blinking lights, juke-box jingles, plastic snow, frantic shoppers, televised solicitation. A little over a week later the celebration of Christ's nativity (followed, I knew, by Mao Tse-tung's seventy-seventh birthday the next day) gave way to New Year's Eve, and 1970 was no more.

Waiting for Ed, I splashed in southern pools under Hollywood skies, dressed up for expensive northern restaurants, lunched on cracked crab at Sausalito bars. Struck by the genuine niceness of my fellow citizens, I was, on the other hand, uneasy at their insularity, their unblissful ignorance, when contradictions, unrest, apprehension, were visible everywhere. A Mill Valley home's plate-glass view framed the lights of San Francisco's bay, where Alcatraz lay like a silent shark in shadow—home, for that moment, of dispossessed Indians. Berkeley University's Sather Gate resounded to the harangues of Jesus freaks and chanting Hari Krishna converts who, swathed in pink and white sheets, their feet gray from pavement pollution, offered paper plates of organically grown raw vegetables and grains.

The rattle of violence formed background to lives hung up on charge-account plates, time payments, drop-out youths on drugs, and competition with the neighbors' clothes and cars. Pieces on sexual crimes headlined home-town newspapers picked up from clipped lawns in the evenings by weary homemakers. Several blocks away from the pretty college campus a few copies of the Sunday *New York Times* arrived weekly, on following Thursdays, at Stockton's Pacific Avenue "newsdealers" where "bachelor books" (pornographic paperbacks) were the owners' main livelihood. Television, larded with deodorizing commercials, occupied me to an extreme. I got hooked on what my sisters called "bad-news time" which, at six o'clock each evening, follows the primary-colored cartoons and cowboy films.

Across the world Vietnam lay pounded bare, victim of presidential pride, war-profiting industries, and the nation's complacency. Seemingly oblivious to neighbors whose objecting sons had gone to prison or left the country, a majority of families sat down together with the televised sight and sound of Southeast Asia's misery floating over their dinners, ignoring too the significance of formerly uncommitted peasants daily turning Communist under the onslaught of American bombers. Cambodia's Prince Sihanouk had said to me in Peking, "When you return to your country, madame, tell the people there that every time a bomb destroys a peasant dwelling, the United States creates Communists."

I wrote to Ed—when are you coming? His letters arrived —why no word from me? Frustratingly, letters took weeks; in Europe mail to and from China had not been difficult. In March, leaving China much later than he'd intended, Ed went directly to Switzerland. Reunited with him by trans-atlantic telephone, I heard the tiredness in his voice. My return to Switzerland was planned via New York, where I had been told interest in publication of Ed's two long inter-views with Premier Chou En-lai existed at that city's most important daily newspaper. They were already scheduled for publication in many other countries.

"Take care of that if you can," Ed said. "It's important to have them published in the States for wide circulation. But come home soon. I miss you and need your help."

Our son, Christopher, telephoned me a few days later in New York. "Pop's terribly tired, Mom. I've never seen him so tired. Like . . ."

"Like . . . I should come home right away?"

"Yeah," he confirmed, "like that."

I verified the newspaper interest, packed and flew to Switzerland.

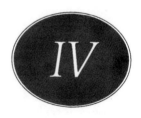

IV

The "boys" (my pre–Women's Liberation way of identifying the male members of the family; habit dies hard) met me at Geneva's air terminal—Chris, slim and fair, taller than his father but very like; Ed, deep brown eyes a twinkling contrast to gray skin and pale hair. Thinner? I wondered. (We had both gained weight on Chinese banquets and unaccustomed nibbling between meals—fresh peanuts, fruits, dates or sweets.) Not much, not *thin*. Overworked, yes. Overextended.

"When we finish the articles we'll find a beach. We'll go to bed at nine and get up when we please. We'll run and swim and sit in Sicilian sun. And *then* we'll write our books."

Hugging the prospect, we sank into the back of the station wagon and let Chris, with shoulders young and strong, drive us home through the late morning.

We entered our village, passed the post office, the

épicerie, the small *auberge,* the winter-iced fountain that
marks the turn into the driveway we share with our next-
door neighbors. The linden looked like a child's drawing
of the biggest tree in the world. How fortunate we were
—the past brimming full, so much still ahead! Snug in
March snow, our farmhouse seemed unexpectedly Chinese
beneath the leaden Swiss sky. It's the stone and the courtyard, I thought, and the sense of having been there for
years. It was also that I had finally been to China and
marked the similarities.

The only people we wanted to see for a while were
friends enough not to casually drop in; when an evening
freed itself for company we'd call them up. A drive along
the winding Begnins road brought us a few hours of relaxa-
tion at Ursula and Harris Russell's home in the foothills of
the Juras; a hop over the countryside a visit with Joan
Jaeger in the old house she lives in, similar to our own, two
kilometers across the fields. Hers has an elegance ours does
not, in spite of do-it-yourself renovation in both, but she
is adept at everything from electrical wiring to needlepoint
and refinishing antiques. Hence the difference. Joan, whose
former husband, Karl Jaeger, created the International
School of America, which did so much to change our lives,
came over from the States with us for that "one year"
fourteen years ago when her children were toddlers and,
like us, stayed on. Blond and slim as a teen-ager, she returns to Ohio now and then for a family reunion, but her
transplanted roots hold strong in Switzerland, supported
by self-reliance, ski poles and recently a handsome horse.
The Russells, too, are "emigrants"—a European-American
combination flourishing in the pleasant peace of the Swiss

countryside with arms outstretched to other worlds and peoples. With them, since good fortune brought us together, we have picnicked, played and puzzled over world events.

As the days went by, the news that was apparently not "fit to print" remained unpublished in the American daily press. An abrupt phone call from New York awakened us at two o'clock one morning to reject the Chou En-lai interviews "for lack of space." It's one of the few times I ever saw Ed *really* angry. We gave up hope of prominent newspaper coverage in the United States; the pieces subsequently appeared with quiet dignity in the *New Republic*, where articles by Edgar Snow had been welcome in the past.

Needled by deadlines and as fast as Ed wrote (his squiggles and arrows as familiar as shorthand to me), I typed the articles due *Epoca* magazine, the Milan weekly that had sponsored the trip to China. It was early to bed at each day's end, shutters closed against the cold, thoughts on work as we went to sleep curled together in our big bed. Village nights can be the same most anywhere.

Ping-pong was the signal. How subtle the Chinese! Write a Hollywood script with *that* story before those little balls began to bounce and nobody would have bought it: that long-haired American youth with peace badges and flowers embroidered on his blue jeans; that sweet-faced teen-ager whose mother might have been quaking at the thought of her daughter being in China; Chou En-lai shaking hands with the U.S. table-tennis team in Peking's main and splendid gymnasium (where Ed had first presented me to the Premier months before at a ping-pong match between China and North Korea); the cheering from the stands as the People's Republic of China met the United States of America across the green of a ping-pong table! We turned on the battered television set we inherited from a neighbor who had returned to New Guinea, and watched the refreshing scene.

With the bounce of international table-tennis balls, our Swiss telephone came alive like the United Nations' switchboard. Joan Jaeger leaped over to handle the calls and messages. It was exciting for her to be part of the action; it was a load off our shoulders to have her help. Monsieur Longchamps, the genial postmaster, delivered telegrams day and night; a lot of people were ready to go to Peking and the only person they knew who knew how to do that was suddenly an old friend. Ed eventually had a form letter printed stating he had no influence on the matter of visas to the People's Republic.

Ed and I had been working steadily, he on Cultural Revolutionary China, I on revolutionary Peking opera and ballet. (My book contract—the first in my life—had been a "birthday present" from Ed before we left for Peking in July 1970. Preparation for this trip had occupied us to the eve of departure. When Ed handed me an envelope along with a glass of champagne the night we acknowledged my increased age, I assumed it was a check; there had been no time to select a personal gift. Inside was a contract for a book on Chinese theatre. Panicking at the sight, I cried, "No! I can't *do* that!" "Try," said Ed seriously, "see if you can." Shortly before he died he read over the almost finished manuscript. "It's good." He grinned. "I knew you'd make it.") With the evident sign from Peking, couched in the mid-April invitation to the U.S. sports team, Ed decided to publish part of the five-hour conversation he had had with Mao Tse-tung in December 1970.

Tang Wen-sheng (known as Nancy Tang), the young, exceptionally bright woman who, when the People's Republic joined the United Nations and, later, during the American presidential pilgrimage to Peking, flashed across national television screens in her role as interpreter, had arrived at our hotel one early morning, catching us both in unusually late sleep. We had been working on notes deep into the night before; at five o'clock, after tossing restlessly, Ed had taken a sedative. If anything could have awakened him, it was Nancy's announcement: "Somebody wants to see you." It did, but he had to fight that pill.

"Chairman Mao said to come as you are," Nancy told Ed. "No formality. Come for breakfast."

"But not in my pajamas!" Ed stumbled sleepily into the big bathroom and splashed water on his face while I found underwear in the cupboard, dove for shoes under the bed.

"Well, no," Nancy laughed. "But just slacks and a sweater. And a warm coat; it's cold outside."

I waited alone in the hotel, that morning Ed went off to see the Chairman. When he returned to our rooms five and a half hours later, I had filled the ashtrays with cigarette stubs, consumed two thermos bottles of tea, and dug up a new cassette knowing he'd want to record his impressions of the meeting. I tried to be patient while we ordered some beer and lunch in our room—then I gasped, "*What* did he SAY!" We ate and talked (the cassette is musical with the tinkle of silver and plates) and by the time Ed had said everything he could remember, he was so sleepy he had to go to bed.

Ed had been told by the Chairman that Richard Nixon would be welcome to come to China, either as a tourist or as President—he could just get on a plane and come. We had held this news for months, waiting for the right time and place to reveal it publicly. *Life* magazine agreed to publish Ed's interview with Mao Tse-tung and an article on his talks with Chou En-lai; the word was out and the subsequent chain of events is history. The week Richard Nixon went to Peking, Ed died in our rambling old farmhouse in the tiny Swiss village of Eysins, Vaud. The date was February 15, 1972.

After ping-pong shook the world in April 1971, we drove to Sperlonga, above Naples on the Italian coast. Our first vacation alone together in years, we casually accepted it as one of many to follow. Fatigue disappeared in salt air and warm sand. Off season, the little town led an undisturbed existence: fishing boats speckled the water; solemn-faced women, in black from head to toe, paraded to and from a soap-sudded backwash of sea, balancing huge baskets of family laundry on their heads; a nucleus of resident hippies prepared a terrace restaurant for the summer tourists who would soon arrive to churn up the now almost deserted beach. Our *albergo* was empty except for a young English couple and their sunbaked little boys. Together we climbed with them over the wave-pounded ruins of Tiberius' summer palace at the far end of the beach, the parents holding on to the two children bent on entering the remains of the Romans' crocodile pond, full of brackish water and the ghosts of condemned slaves. Middays, Signor Italio and his family served newly caught fish and homemade pasta covered with native tomatoes and herbs. I had never tasted fresh mozzarella before; they showed us the Italian way of eating it—peppered, salted, dribbled with olive oil. It was delicious.

We napped after lunch and returned to the beach until the sun dimmed. Ed swam too far out in the lonely sea, causing me to rage like a wet Rumpelstiltskin, leaping up and down, yelling on the shoreline. It was not the first time he had terrified me by bobbing about in the distant blue. Ed always balanced a lightness of risk-taking with conscientious responsibility, and he possessed a need of investigation with a buoyancy of spirit which, through our life together, made me marvel that after each hazardous experience he somehow managed to show up again. Indeed, I could hardly believe that he had *been* there, years ago, across the crowded room of the New York City cocktail party at which we had first met, I as a young actress, he a mature foreign correspondent. Somewhere within, he had a sense of self-preservation that kept him on the safe side of a danger line, but I often felt it was tenuous protection—as when the dot of his head melted into the horizon of a sea or river or lake, which almost always happened when he plunged into irresistible water. Many materials formed the fabric of his character; daring-to-do is noticeable in the weave. I had read *Red Star Over China* long before I met the author; it should have been no surprise that he played as intensely as he worked, inconsiderate of conventional cautions.

Wives of foreign correspondents have to have strong

nerves and patience to accept their husbands' long ab-
sences, sometimes dangerous travel, frustrating periods of
being out of touch. When I married Ed he was over the
most hectic part of his career, but I knew life with him
would be neither sedentary nor simple. Returned from
war years of reporting the upheavals of Nazi-ravaged
Russia and battle-smashed Europe, he had, before that,
mule-backed through poppy-planted, bandit-infested areas
of China, witnessed massacres and mass famines, covered insurrection and civil war and, smuggled in and out
of enemy-barricaded "Red China," had made the Chinese
revolution as readable as an epic novel.

He was no typical American to me, with my background
of convent classrooms, country-club proms, college-frater-
nity dates, wartime stage-door canteen duty-dancing between matinée and evening performances, and the rarefied
life of Broadway's backstage, yet Ed personified those ele-
ments we Americans prize as typical and he put into daily
practice what many pay lip service to on Sundays. I knew
the man well before we married. I loved his gentleness as
much as his courage, his sense of humor as much as his wisdom, his independent thinking as much as his regard for
facts, his objectivity as much as his involvement. I became
accustomed to his forgetfulness, his scattered clothes, I ad-
justed to his lateness (theatre trained me to be prompt)
and was constantly struck by his sensibility to fellow human beings. I was touched by his directness as well as his
subtleness, his strength as well as his sensitivity. Delighted
by his curiosity, I'd agree to turning off a direct road to
investigate probable shortcuts, and then get furious when
we arrived an hour late for a dinner party and were met by

anxious hosts. Admiring his do-it-yourself tinkering with electricity (he had been a proper eagle scout), I'd still have a fit when he nearly electrocuted himself. Appreciative of the tennis game he enjoyed so much, I'd scold when he played too long in the midday sun. But I had no mixed feelings when he resigned as associate editor of the *Saturday Evening Post* in 1951 rather than lend his name to an editorial policy he disapproved, or when he went to the defense of falsely accused men and women knowing the risk of blacklisting and debt—both of which came. Above all, I am glad he returned from the wars and we met that summer night several decades ago, even if some of the hairs on my head became prematurely gray when, as at Sperlonga, I awaited his return from the sea.

At night on that Italian vacation we dressed up for village promenade (I wore the floppy straw hat Ed had bought me at the street market), licked pastel ice cream cones in the seaside square or drank sooty-black, sugared coffee at a café high up over the Mediterranean where a Saracen tower rises gloomily to the sky. Ed bumped into a visiting Italian citizen who had removed himself permanently to New York and invited him for a drink at the hotel. The straw-hatted gentleman politely begged off from the drink ("delicate stomach"), took us instead on a tour of the tomato fields, and filled us in on not only the whole town population—he was related to most of them—but at least a quarter of the Bronx as well. And his stomach. I had other interests and dodged him each day when I went to buy the English-language paper up from Rome. Ed enjoyed his company. "Nice fellow," he maintained. "Interesting." Most human beings were to Ed.

Two weeks was all we could spare from work. On the way home through the soft Italian spring we stopped outside Florence to visit Oliver Clubb, son of our long-time friends, Mariann and Edmund; Oliver, like his father, is an experienced political scientist. The junior Clubbs were in residence handling courses for the University of Syracuse year-in-Europe. Emmy was keeping the house and Florence going, their little girls were attending school, mixing Italian with English, and when otherwise unoccupied, flying around the huge tree in front of the house on a contraption that resembled a combined merry-go-round, flying saucer and swing. Ed and I both wanted to join the whirl but it wouldn't bear our weights; we settled for walks through the olive groves and lots of talk in the sprawly house. Oliver and Ed took pictures whenever they weren't in conversation serious enough to make them forget their cameras. The photographs Oliver took of Ed belie the existence of disease; with a suntanned face and a camera case slung over one shoulder, he looks like a healthy, relaxed vacationer. The malady was deep down; even then, if we had suspected something drastically wrong, it would have been too late.

Summer arrived quickly after we returned to Switzerland; work schedules were disturbed by the speed of international developments. The months following ping-pong and the Nixon announcement of an impending trip to Peking produced constant requests for information and interviews with Ed, the sudden flow of correspondence was taxing. But sometimes we gardened—a pleasure Ed had brought into my life; there was lettuce, tomatoes, strawberries, beans, and the good young American corn that Europeans still don't quite understand but is our midsummer delight—and sometimes we danced, sillily, by ourselves. I remember a final fling of exuberance, brought on by a favorite dance record played loud on the phonograph, that left us middle-agedly panting and exhausted from fun. Ed reacted to rhythm like the musician he had thought he might become when he was the proud teen-age owner of a saxophone, instinctively and with the improvisation of a child, though his style leaned on Shanghai circa 1930 and I was sometimes aware that arm-pumping in crowded dance areas might have led to bloody noses. I adore dancing and am uninhibited on our living-room floor.

By August, Mary Heathcote joined us from New York. Ed's editor since 1957, Mary had become as close as a member of our family; she had stayed with us before to work side by side one of her most favorite authors while he in turn sighed with relief, knowing that her perceptive judgment and easy relationship meant work in depth with facility and calm. Mary also meant a good time for all concerned. Now she appeared, balanced between two crutches, nursing a broken foot. (The tap-tap-tap of Mary's sticks remained an established refrain through the rest of the summer and on until autumn turned to winter cold and Mary left, in December, bidding a broken-hearted good-bye.)

When at night Ed became plagued by insomnia, I'd wake to hear the sticks, the clink of kitchenware, the murmured voices; I knew Mary had joined him downstairs for hot milk or tea, was taking notes as he talked, or simply storing what he said in her drowsy head. I knew, too, that she'd stay up with him until he was able to rest again. They worked together, the two of them, in unusual unity.

Ed became more and more tired. So did I. I was soon to discover I had hepatitis, but at this point it was simply weariness to me. Mary's foot got better, not enough to discard the crutches, though she graduated to a less obtrusive pair than the telephone poles she had on arrival. The three of us ached at the end of each day from hours of typing. We'd laugh at each other's moans and groans, sometimes exaggerated, sometimes not. Our Swiss family doctor, Robert Panchaud, pumped us with vitamins, recommended massage and repose, put Mary through special therapy at the small hospital, X-rayed Ed's back, told us to stop smoking, endured our broken French and was always the "doll" we told him he was. This came out as *"poupée,"* and though he didn't understand the application of that word to himself, he knew we meant something nice.

From the first winter of our residence at St. Cergue ten years before, tall Dr. Panchaud and later his tiny doctor wife, Andrée, have been our dearest Swiss friends. At that time we had rented an old stone-walled house perched on a roll of hill above a small ski slope in the Jura Mountains. St. Cergue, grown up over centuries near the Swiss-French border (direct route to Paris some five hundred kilometers distant—I loved seeing the sign pointing through the woods to "gay Paree"), is high enough above Lac Leman to command, when there is no fog, a breathtaking view of the two countries—Geneva on the Swiss side, sparkling sedately on crisp, clear nights, and Mont Blanc in France, gleaming in the sun like a giant ice-cream sundae. During those first years away from the United

States, every time that mound of snow emerged from the mist I felt a nostalgic pang for hot fudge.

After a casual term in the mountaintop primary class, Christopher and Sian had started more advanced public school below on the lake, daily taking the little red train (the Toonerville Trolley, we called it) down and back up the mountain. Dr. Panchaud came up, too, from Nyon twice a week to tend the resident population and transient guests, the latter mostly ski casualties. We soon learned he'd come whenever a doctor was urgently needed—at three o'clock in the morning if an appendix screamed or a child's ear hurt enough to frighten a sleepy parent. He was comfort and joy, our Dr. Panchaud, a devoted country doctor of that "old school" one hears about but seldom encounters any more. The children and I spent snowed-in winters at St. Cergue while Ed traveled to China, the United States, and near and far. I enjoyed being among the dark-green firs which in the distance above the village ski slope looked like the little ones we used to buy at the ten-cent store for the Christmas crèche, their branches glistening with sprayed-on silver. It was never lonely. Joan was close by—actually it was she who had discovered the piny paradise before we moved up—and a group of appealing wanderers made up what was known as the "foreign colony." This comprised a fair sampling of nationalities, considering the size of St. Cergue: Australians, New Guineans, English, Spanish, Canadians, Indians, Americans, one Hungarian, and a couple of German and French families who had become virtually Swiss. For us the numbers were augmented by guests, expected and un-, who wound their way to our house when they learned that

Edgar Snow was in residence. For three years we lived in a house that had belonged to Henri Bergson; our status was double-pronged, but it surprised Ed that *he* would be sought out. The eminence of Bergson had long been established and the village was proud of their adopted son. But when Ed's book about his 1960 trip to China came out, copies were placed in the windows of St. Cergue's butcher shop, grocery store, and the sports shop across the street that bears the sign "WE SPEAK BROKEN ENGLISH," and we felt we too had found a place of esteem in our village. Some who took the trouble to seek Ed out include present-day good friends; Lee Ambrose is high on that list. Lee plowed through snow drifts to our front door; we have enjoyed her company ever since. Editor and indefatigable traveler, she applies common sense to worldly conflicts, and her precise mind includes an understanding of mathematics which she occasionally coupled with Ed's at a casino just across the border in France. Ed almost always lost his hundred francs, Lee usually tripled hers, while I, mathematically deficient, roamed from gaming table to gaming table feeling as if I were an extra in an old Bogart film.

I also had the children and their growing band of *camarades*. Sian and Chris returned each evening from school, always famished, in spite of a hot and hearty Swiss lunch, for bananas, peanut butter, milk, and an hour later, a complete American dinner.

"After all *that* food?" I'd ask, astonished.

"Mom, we're *starving*. *We* work!"

I suppose it looked to them as if I didn't, but besides taking care of a stream of visitors, I taught English at the small private school, pounded away at French and the typewriter, knitted kilometers of sweaters and read as I had not done in years—a lot on China, strengthening a foundation that was to serve me in good stead in the future. It was Dr. Panchaud, dropping by for chats on the sun porch after village medical visits, who encouraged me to take up skiing, who helped untangle French verbs, recommended regional wines, deciphered *Le Monde,* and told stories of the town personalities, some of whose families seemed to go back as far as St. Cergue's beginnings—and that was before the Roman Empire. When Ed stayed home long enough, he and Robert quickly found companionship. For ten years the Panchauds and the Snows have remained close.

When we later purchased the Eysins farmhouse in the valley by the lake, we became near neighbors and Robert a steady controller of the family's health, supervising colds, sore throats and various household bugs. He knows how to care and, conscientious as a saint, turns to others if symptoms indicate a matter outside his scope.

Puzzled by Ed's growing discomfort, our good doctor insisted on examinations by specialists. The tests indicated no seriousness or emergency (cancer roots itself cunningly), and a proposed hospitalization for further medical exploration was postponed to a later, more convenient moment. Ed accepted the pain as a nuisance ("lumbago," "arthritis") and we soothed each other by the promise of another checkup and more rest when time allowed.

In those days of heightened pressure, disease took over in the guise of normality: we were *used* to fatigue when writing schedules consumed many hours of a long day;

aches are *expected* by authors glued to typewriter chairs. So I massaged Ed's back, he mine, lying out on the warm garden grass; we jogged for exercise early mornings and I was only vaguely upset when empty aspirin bottles had to be replaced more frequently than before.

Three things happened in October.

The People's Republic of China entered the United Nations against the stubborn opposition of the United States and with the excited approbation of a good majority of the total membership. Mary, Ed and I had a drink on that. Then an autumn afternoon brought publisher Timo Kärnekull with his about-to-be-released Swedish edition of *Red Star Over China* to our house. As the world is well aware, the Swedes have a particular way with color and design; Timo had produced a beauty of a book. With him was Nils Gunnar Nilson, photographing as we talked. Not only are his pictures a record of a pleasant day, they mark a turning of time, for copies arrived from Stockholm not long after and from them I saw with a stab that Ed was gravely ill. It was there in his eyes, recorded on the photographs. Acceptance was impossible ("You *exaggerate*," I scolded myself); the moment passed, outside on our terrace where I had gone alone to read the mail. Sweeping away shock, I clamped an agonized denial over the knowledge and turned quickly toward the life about me, the unseasonably sunny garden, the chattering birds, the deceptive warmth of October sun. And yet it's cold, I thought, shivering.

The third event occurred in hazy unreality. I had become increasingly listless, groping through a day, feeling "flu-y," forcing exertion. We talked of a rest; I was too tired to react. When Ed returned from Geneva one late afternoon with a ten-day round-trip ticket to Morocco on the next day's plane, I couldn't believe he'd go. Near tears, worried, I helped him pack. He wanted to go at once, and though upset that I felt unwell, he knew Mary was there to help. He put our two manuscripts in his suitcase along with summer shorts, swimming trunks, and changes of shirts and socks. "I need sun and sea and I need to be alone for a time," he told me, and I let him go then without argument. He was in search of the peace that had come earlier in the spring on the Italian shore.

I was in bed, sicker, when he returned. His face was bronzed and lined. His back had been better when packed into warm sand, he said, but he hadn't slept much at night. Days had been spent on the shore playing chess with an American student, using the beach as a chessboard and shells for the men. Ed had worked on his book, made important notes in mine, and, it turned out after he emptied his suitcase, had left both scripts in Morocco. A cablegram produced the two—brought by the young American chess partner who, receiving the S O S just as he was leaving, detoured to Eysins, stayed for a meal, and flew off to Rome, his original destination. I was too ill to meet him, I don't even recall his name, but I appreciate his marvelous response to our emergency and place him high among those who pay attention to human need.

Ed took me to the hospital in late November. Feeling miserable, I snuggled into care, glad to be rid of telephones and callers. A pansy-blue-eyed floor head nurse with the happy name of Mademoiselle Bonjour controlled things with gentle efficiency, and the regular day nurse swooped in and out of my room like a mother swallow. Hospital briskness was softened by a lovely Scandinavian youngster, Lisa, whose English sounded like the murmur of fjord waters and whose generous attention made me, in weakness, want to cry. From Lisa came the extra cup of tea, the sunny smile, the whispered "Good night." From the kindly chief internist came necessary poking, prodding and blood tests. Diagnosis: infectious hepatitis. There was nothing to do but rest in bed, stick to a special diet and wait to recover. Soon I turned bright-yellow. *"Jaunisse"* they call it lyrically in French. It sounded nicer to me than jaundice.

Ed and I speculated that he, too, might have the same debilitating disease; his fatigue was the same as mine. He reluctantly joined me in the spacious double room, piled the tables and chairs with books and papers, and submitted impatiently to a variety of tests. He had no time for hospitals; he was there only to be dismissed. The doctors seemed guarded (the dreadful photo came to my mind), and danger signals, discreetly disguised by professional manners, flashed in warning. I shoved fear down, pulling my sickness close as protection.

Learning that both his parents were in the hospital, Chris, who had started school in London, returned home. He didn't say "What's the matter?" or "I'm worried about you," but he was there and we were glad.

Ed smoked too much, slept badly and paced the hallway at night, to the nurses' concern. One morning, determined to finish his book in less cramped style, he up and left the hospital before I awoke.

"He's like a tiger in a cage," the nurses said.

"He's gravely ill, madame." The doctor's eyes were solemn, sympathetic. "His liver is very enlarged."

"How big?"

"King-sized."

It was not hepatitis. It was cancer of the pancreas which had by now deeply affected the liver. A specialist was immediately consulted, an operation scheduled, and though nobody said it out loud, there seemed to be a big "if" . . .

Not until later was I told that a young medical technician had remarked privately, after scanning the preoperative tests, that if they had been his father's, he would have rejected surgery—it was too late, too painful, and in his opinion, to no avail. Nobody put it to us this way. I do not know what our choice would have been if they had.

The night I learned of the seriousness of the disease I borrowed a cigarette from the nurse on duty, my first since falling ill. Sooner than the doctors counseled, I went home. Ed said no, wait longer, but I knew I couldn't.

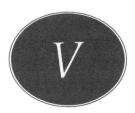

Ed entered the hospital in Lausanne the day after a double birthday celebration with a lopsided chocolate cake and a bottle of wine. Chris, turned twenty-two, shared the honors with Mary—who wasn't telling. Over the familiar flicker of the candlelit cake we rendered an off-tune "Happy Birthday to You" and lingered around the table just long enough to savor the fleeting moments.

Since I had been back home only a few days and was still too shaky to drive a car, Joan took Ed to the hospital the next morning. It was better, as she could be perky and bright and kid about his load of typewriter, books and papers. We made sure it included a toothbrush and Ed's inevitably misplaced reading glasses—the only pair we could find at the last minute was the one hinged together with a paper clip. I waved the car out of sight from the upstairs window and fell wearily back into bed, unable to sleep, unable to stay on my feet.

By Friday afternoon, final medical examinations were completed, the date set for surgery the following Tuesday. Worn and weary, Ed came home for a weekend of paper work in his studio. On Saturday morning he talked to the neighbors next door, Monsieur and Madame Granger, leaning over the fence that separates our garden from their fruit orchard, to chat of crops and weather and, I suppose, of life and death. Such things make normal conversation for country people. Close to eighty, this modest Swiss couple know a lot from faces. Their own showed concern as they moved slowly away, turning to wave at their gate. Through the weeks that followed we were to eat Madame's oven-hot fruit tarts (left unobtrusively on the kitchen table), and they were to share the moist, tender "chiao tze," the spice-pungent chicken and crisp spring rolls Ambassador Chen and his wife later carried in quantity from the Chinese embassy in Bern or the Geneva consulate staff brought over to tempt Ed's appetite. East met West with ease in our tiny community, the villagers accepting the Chinese strangers as bearers of unusual love for "les Américains."

The night before the operation, Chris and I left a subdued but normal-looking Ed, pajama-clad and relaxed from a pill, sitting in a plastic-leather armchair with newspapers, books, radio and phone at fingers' touch, in the hospital high above the choppy lake and night-bound, empty streets. The room seemed almost cozy after we had mussed it up a bit. Chris and I returned the next morning to find it sterile, empty of bed and occupant, irrevocably changed.

How does one know the truth? I was numb with fatigue and worry, but after the four-hour operation, hope revived.

A Death with Dignity

It was over, it had been long, but as with a jury out for a considerable length of time, the verdict could be good. When Ed was wheeled back to the room, moaning with pain, his eyes open and glazed, his face pasty-gray, there was no indication from the attendants, occupied with drains and needles; when the doctors emerged from unseen places, they were gravely polite and evasive: the chief surgeon was performing another operation—I would see him later. I was shocked by the stark postoperative mechanics; close to fainting, I was led from the room and given a cup of tea.

As a little girl, Sian used to draw pictures that all children draw. I remembered a colored one of two black-bearded, button-eyed purple creatures sitting with their crossed legs entangled, a funnel of curly smoke rising above their heads. A child's conception of adult inscrutability emanated from the pair. Sian, age five, explained: "They are doctors who cross their legs and talk about important things." Now I felt all that was in that long-ago picture: there was nothing concrete to get hold of from the enigmatic real human beings. It evidently wasn't that good after all but no one pronounced a sentence. And did I really want one if it wasn't good? Would Ed? Would knowing be too painful? All I could grasp was a future obscure, an Ed too sick to be coherent, and an implied expectation that I be undemanding. I didn't press for details. It was as if posing questions meant being uncooperative and everyone seemed so occupied that I was hesitant to intrude, but an inner coldness thickened inside and when Mary had to go home three days after the operation (her mother was ill in the States), some of the shoved-aside truth finally burst out. I sobbed in her arms until nothing was left but exhaustion. Without being told, we both realized that it was only a question of time. Mary went off and I knew full well how hard it was for her to leave.

There is point to dwelling on those hospital days and the nightmare nights at home as each day passed in anxiety; our later experience showed this should not have been, but for us they were about the best conditions one could *buy* anywhere in the United States or Western Europe. A private Swiss clinic provides external comforts and modern facilities that must rate as luxurious in comparison to many Western equivalents; one can purchase amenities and physical decencies that blunt the sharp rupture of normal life forced into hospital restriction and at a far lesser cost than in the United States. Even for a foreigner the toll, including room service, phone, etc., for Ed's stay in a private room with bath, was a fraction of the price it would have been at home.

Beyond ability to pay, which can be decisive in terms of the quality of technical treatment, there is the quality of overall care of the ill, and that is largely up to individuals in charge—how, out of rationed time and personal understanding of service, they dispense their controlled emotions, sympathy, unique contributions. Most people are not prepared for the ordeal of dying, or even of being seriously sick. Practicing physicians, many of them, encased in their special worlds, dole out information and communication cautious of cost and risk. Every case demands involvement and distance; one gives of oneself measuredly, else the individual, coping with constant and countless pressures, has no more to give. Training has been centered on technique and mechanics; experience has led to self-protection and restraint. The human being has become an instrument. Wholeness of relationship can come only when a society organizes the means—ideological, educational, physical—that provide people with the circumstances and the will to behave in communal effort in full commitment.

In her book *Question and Answers on Death and Dying,* Dr. Elisabeth Kübler-Ross,* a Chicago psychiatrist, recounts the experiment she helped conduct among terminally ill patients in a Chicago hospital in 1965. Below the book's title are the words: "What the dying have to teach doctors, nurses, clergy and their own families." I wish I had read it before the fact of dying changed our own lives. She writes:

> . . . dying nowadays is more gruesome in many ways, namely, more lonely, mechanical, and dehumanized; at times it is even difficult to determine technically when the time of death has occurred.
>
> Dying becomes lonely and impersonal because the patient is often taken out of his familiar environment and rushed to an emergency room. Whoever has been very sick and has required rest and comfort especially may recall his experience of being put on a stretcher and enduring the noise of the ambulance siren and hectic rush until the hospital gates open. Only those who have lived through this may appreciate the discomfort and cold necessity of such transportation which is only the beginning of a long ordeal—hard to endure when you are well, difficult to express in words when noise, light, pumps, and voices are all too much to put up with. It may well be that we might consider more the patient under the sheets and blankets and perhaps stop our well-

* New York: Macmillan, 1969.

meant efficiency and rush in order to hold the patient's hand, to smile, or to listen to a question . . . Is this approach our own way to cope with and repress the anxieties that a terminally or critically ill patient evokes in us? Is our concentration on equipment, on blood pressures, our desperate attempt to deny the impending death which is so frightening and discomforting to us that we displace all our knowledge onto machines, since they are less close to us than the suffering face of another human being which would remind us once more of our lack of omnipotence, our own limits and failures, and last but not least perhaps our own mortality?

While reading this, I thought of China, of its physical sights and sounds. It struck me that I had seen but never heard ambulances there. Emergencies are taken care of without the shrieks of sirens.

I was completely unready for the actuality of terminal illness. So, I believe, was Ed. Dying wasn't presented to him openly in the beginning, and he didn't (openly) accept the hints of it. I registered them but stuffed them away like something obscene. Our inability to accept *our* mortality unbalanced us.

Never a patient patient, in that he resented the resultant loss of time and activity, Ed had been in and out of hospitals much more often than I, perhaps because of insufficient diet during the war years abroad as a journalist, perhaps from hidden germs picked up through prolonged travel in tropical and poverty-stricken areas, dormant until he worked his body too hard. Not that he was sickly, far from it; he was full of an energy and vitality that made him even more exasperated with temporary immobility.

On my part, I reassured myself that, after all, we had the

best that money could buy—I think we did—but I couldn't fathom the confusion that resulted as daily I muddled through implications, ambiguities, indirection and—expectancy, for there was hope of some sort, it seemed, and we clung to that until the unexpectedly rapid course of the disease took it away.

I was dissatisfied with what I heard, or did not hear, right after the operation from the affable assistant surgeon, whose solicitude, a comfort of sorts as he talked, lost its strength after he left. I telephoned his superior for information and was told quite firmly not to interrupt his office consultation hours. I waited for him in the main lobby of the hospital, catching him as he strode in from the street—he was polite, considerate, and in a hurry.

I tried to understand the charts that substituted for communication; I held back worries, guarded anxiety, kept attentively available in the corridor outside the line of closed doors. There were others with me in the hallway—an Italian wife, a young husband, a middle-aged mother. We became partners in waiting, fused together in apprehension cloaked by tentative cordialities, exchanging uncertain "Good nights" when we left our sick at day's end to try to reenter the world that continued outside. I wondered who was behind each of the impersonal white doors, interiors glimpsed by a fraction when lunch trays were wheeled in or doctors entered with stethoscope and paraphernalia. Overnight a room would empty, be open to a morning view of withered flowers and thumbed magazines thrust in bins as blue-gowned cleaners scrubbed and aired and sterilized for another occupant. Had the patient gone home? Or died? I blotted out imagined scenes. A known figure from the corridor group would be replaced by a taut new face that slowly became part of the days of waiting. I wouldn't know them today if we passed on the street, except perhaps the Italian wife because her face reminded me of someone I love. When she gave way to tears once, silently in a corner, huddled forlornly in her full-length mink coat, I wanted to put out my arms and share our grief. But I didn't. I too was restricted.

I had a quarrel with a cool, self-contained nurse who acted like a prison matron bent on keeping order and who regarded me as a nuisance from that moment when I had almost fainted at the sight and sound of Ed immediately after the operation. She dealt with his cries and moans as if he were a naughty child: "Mr. Snow, *behave* yourself!" Novice to the treatment of the critically ill, I held back instinctive protest, but my worry showed and so did the nurse's reaction—she had no time to be bothered. After we tangled over what was to her another minor matter, she found out that I was just out of a hospital and not really ready yet to be, and I discovered that she had recently been ill herself; long and busy hours too quickly resumed had given her a case of jangled nerves contained by distant manner, revealed by flairs of irritation. Once we knew this about each other, I became less antagonistic and she, in an attempt at compatibility, even brought herself to smile a time or two at Ed's jokes in his funny French. I suppose she had problems at home. They were a mystery to me, and mine were of no concern to her. She was working for a pay check; she wasn't putting in overtime to give extra attention.

This, of course, had been her training. The idealistic,

dedicated women who enter the nursing profession are forced into molds of behavior that more often than not produce subservience and a detachment that borders on boredom.

> . . . nurses of every rank from aide up are just "ancillary workers" in relation to the doctors (from the Latin *ancilla,* maid servant). From the nurses' aide, whose menial tasks are spelled out with industrial precision, to the "professional" nurse, who translates the doctors' orders into the aide's tasks, nurses share the status of uniformed maid service to the dominant male professionals. . . . Nurses are taught not to question, not to challenge. "The doctor knows best." He is the shaman, in touch with the forbidden, mystically complex world of Science which we have been taught is beyond our grasp. Women health workers are alienated from the scientific substance of their work, restricted to the "womanly" business of nurturing and housekeeping—a passive, silent majority.*

Thus the division continues: the doctor treating the illness apart from the patient, the patient nursed by workers whose interests are impersonal, the family standing by, caught in ignorance and worry.

Rounds finished each evening, heading for home (or another hospital?), the tired surgeon stopped to take my hand to half answer a rehearsed, carefully compressed question as we walked together down the hallway to the elevator. The doors would open, slide shut across his

* From the introduction to *Witches, Midwives, and Nurses: A History of Women Healers,* by Barbara Ehrenreich and Deirdre English (Glass Mountain Pamphlets, P.O. Box 238, Oyster Bay, N.Y. 11771. Reprinted in 1973 by Black & Red, Box 9546, Detroit, Mich. 48202).

wrinkled white coat, and I'd wait again another day. One evening I asked him once more if I could arrange a visit to his office during regular hours to discuss matters before hospitalization ended. We had been told the stay would be ten days maximum; upon insistence (mine), the period had been slightly extended, and as the final days drew near I felt Ed was still too ill and I too inexperienced to take care of him. A livable-with, live-in nurse seemed as hard to obtain as a gold-plated one.

"Madame," spluttered the doctor in a crackle of tension, "if I gave *everybody* in the hospital as much time as I give *you,* I would have no *time* for *anybody!*"

He wheeled off, braked himself with physical effort, turned back to say, "We'll see . . . we'll see," pulled open the next patient's door (the Italian's) and entered into someone else's troubles. We never had the talk.

Again I forced myself to try to understand: he is not a mean man, this specialized surgeon of forty-odd years. His professional reputation is undeniable, his responsibilities are too many, his obligations too taxing, his time too limited, and his work too often keeps him uncomfortably occupied with the heartbroken. He meets the magnitude of the demands made as best he can, conscientious, no doubt, but remote, strained, tense. I wouldn't like to be him—or his wife.

A ringing echo sounded in the midst of this: during my years as an actress I had played a neurotic nurse in a television soap opera about hospital life. (We actors found the operating scenes great fun and horseplayed them to our high amusement during rehearsals. On camera we appeared as professional as Dr. Kildare himself.) The ups and downs of make-believe doctors and nurses attracted an afternoon audience of millions five days a week. A hospital provides absorbing drama—who doesn't empathize when the unknown child falls in a well? In reality these characters, caught up in the highly charged situations found in soap serials, do exist behind all the walls of all the hospitals all over the world. It is much easier to watch such drama unfold on a television screen than to be a participant in actuality, whether as patient, family, or staff, thrust into real-life scenes in which complex individual motivations, rather than an author's pen, bring on selfish struggle and computerized care.

There were many problems, recognizable to those who have sojourned in hospitals anywhere, minor or simply irritating when one is not critically ill, major when one is. Private night nurses, mandatory under our circumstances, were not easily obtainable; hospitals are understaffed and personnel is overworked and often underpaid. We made do with retired nurses who were not efficient, and with supposedly efficient medical students who were tired, arrived late and used the paid opportunity to bone up on forthcoming examinations. Even *day* care was not constantly available during that first critical week; this proved hazardous, though less for us perhaps than for others, as Chris or I was there from morning to night, once we saw that this was a necessity. I often thought about people who have no family or friends nearby, not to speak of little or no money—the underprivileged, the lost, the forgotten (or shelved) aged, the castaways at the mercy of come what, or who, may. The world we know revolves around ability to pay. A mitigating factor is the committed individuals who act with compassion as well as skill, but they are the exceptions and are unsupported by a community.

Once, before I arrived in the morning, Ed had been left alone long enough to get halfway out of bed. I found him, drains and tubes dangling, struggling for his slippers, trying to get out of "this damn hotel and go *home*." In near delirium, he fought needed restraints, and there were times when the nurses' signal light remained unanswered so long that I had to risk dashing out into the corridor for help. It was imperative that he not be left alone, but family presence was the only guarantee that he would not be. I can imagine what would have happened if we had not been there; I have since been told of cases in some hospitals in which people have acquired stitched-up gashes on head or body, though call buttons were available and nurses within earshot. Despite, or because of, the privacy of a single room, I began to wish we had chosen a double, or even a small ward: there, under the eyes of roommates, a patient would be less likely to fall out of bed or fade away as a result of a pulled-out tube.

When pain seemed beyond endurance, it was I who talked a nurse into giving the scheduled shot ahead of the *precise* hour, and I who pleaded not to awaken him when soothing sleep coincided with breakfast, tea or untimely temperature checks that satisfy routine. Some of the nurses and orderlies were cooperative and some were not; their feelings seemed mostly smothered, while mine were raw and exposed. The staff apparently had too many obligations to tolerate nonconformity, though the hospital did not appear to be overly full and desk work or corridor conversations sometimes seemed more demanding than a patient's call. An element of chance marked each day, an unseizable factor determined by unpredictable individuals —*their* weaknesses, strengths, whims, anxieties, *their* grasp of obligation—under an undefined and yet implacable routine, in which surface tension or boredom became infectious. A protective veneer, a toughness, forms over those who accept our institutional conditions. I was not to fully comprehend the reason for its existence until after the Chinese demonstrated that it need not be so, and in this I was remiss; I believe I should have insisted on answers, even provoked attention.

> A Los Angeles doctor offers one dramatic suggestion on how to get attention when needed (although his proximity to Hollywood does give it a certain histrionic quality). "When you can't get anybody to come into your room," he says, "throw a bedpan against the wall. If that fails, fall out of bed. That should bring the whole nursing staff on the run. And a doctor is obliged to examine you immediately." *

A cancer specialist, called in for clinical consultation just before we left the hospital, was an unwitting example of the absence of attention paid. Apprehensive that a person unknown to us, new to the case, might, however innocently, cause Ed alarm at a time when he was unprepared to handle facts starkly put, I sought assurance that the man would be presented as a regular blood technician, that no discussion would take place in front of Ed before I first had the specialist's diagnosis. This had been agreed to and when the somber-faced man arrived long after the ap-

---

* "How to Survive the Hospital," by Thomas Thompson, *Good Housekeeping* (June 1974).

pointed time, I watched him go into Ed's room with the surgeon, dreading the almost inevitably bad report but relieved that it would pass through me to my husband, not through this cold stranger. He emerged fifteen minutes later, looking drawn and tired. As he gave me his report (bad), something made me realize it must be a repetition of what he had said inside the room.

"You didn't tell this to my husband?"

"But of course, madame. Why not?"

"It . . . was *understood* you were to discuss this with me first!"

He blinked, uncertain. "You are Americans. It is well known that in your country the patient is always told."

Blinks again. I froze. "It depends on *how* one is told, monsieur."

Christopher came out of his father's room; he had been inside to translate if the doctor's French had not been understood. It had been understood. Chris said, "I couldn't stop him, Mom. He told Pop everything. It's pretty bad."

I went into the room. Ed's face looked diminished and crinkled, framed by disheveled hair against the white pillows. "There's lots to be done, darling," I said close to him.

"Yes," he murmured, "lots."

I think he was thinking of his obligations, his work, of his unfinished book. In any case, by the next day Ed had reached out on his own, denying the harshness of the doctor's report. He spoke of "lesions" instead of metastasis. And I grasped at straws.

Later, after Ed was out of the hospital, we drove back into the city to see the specialist again. Then he was understanding and attentive. Ed counted enormously on the chemotherapy treatments about to begin. Visibly moved by such determination to live, the doctor did not destroy the hope. Privately he told me he had been so ill himself that other day that he had had to get out of bed to keep the appointment, that no one had told him not to reveal the full facts to the patient at that time. He seemed truly distressed. There, in his office, where he daily deals with hopelessness, he was a sympathetic person—by appointment. If I were to have called upon him for immediate aid after this consultation, it's unlikely that he would have responded personally. He had a crammed agenda, limited hours and a protective answering service.

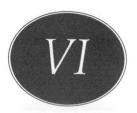

VI

It was Chris who put it frankly one wet night after we had walked over slippery cobblestones to the city parking lot a few blocks from the hospital. I can still see the blurred faces of home-going couples clinging to each other under see-through umbrellas, the bare-headed students waiting for a bus; I can hear chatter, laughter, the click of heels on stone, still smell the meals cooking behind lighted, softly splattered windows. I wished as hard as a child that the four of us could be up in one of those snug rooms, together, healthy, safe.

As we got into the car Chris said that he'd *want* to know if he were dying, that he'd want to *use* the time that was left.

I said, "But if there's *no* time? Or not enough? He's too sick now. Yes, if he *has* time. He's been told; he doesn't want to accept it. We can't force him. We don't even know how long ourselves. *Nobody* seems to know! We must find out what to do!"

The terror of decisions to be made without guidance, without experience, engulfed me. Throughout our marriage Ed and I had made important decisions together, relying on each other. Now he couldn't decide for himself, couldn't really contribute. Words came back from somewhere: "Uninformed choice is not rational choice." They joined in rhythm with the motion of the car: ra-tion-al choice, ra-tion-al choice; I longed to know the wise, the right thing to do. Why *didn't* I—what was wrong? Chris drove on; gusts of wet snow swirled in the headlight glare, as they had before under normal conditions when we had driven home from theatres, from airports, from reunions after partings, from partings when we knew we'd meet again. My son's youth seemed flamboyant, brazenly confident. I felt inept, old, utterly dislocated.

In the hospital corridor I smoked and sometimes stuffed down lumps of cold sandwiches. There was hot soup, meals were available; I couldn't eat. I waited. I waited and I wrote letters—to Ed's family in Boston and Kansas City, to mine in California, to doctor friends in New York, Paris, London, seeking help, asking for something, someone, to save my husband's life. And I wrote to China, hesitatingly, wondering to whom I should write, what I could expect from so far away.

Lee Ambrose decided me. Hearing of our illnesses, she descended from a mountain retreat where she was working on a book. Her dark hair was curly from rain, one hand clutched a florist's spring bouquet as if it had become part of her. It dripped on the floor as she came out of the elevator to say, "Tell me what I can do." I knew at that instant. I addressed a letter to Dr. George Hatem (his Chinese name is Ma Hai-teh), and gave it to Lee to mail special delivery to Peking. Reliable Swiss postal service; reliable tear-blocked Lee. When I brought the flowers in to Ed he smiled wanly. "Give her my love. Tell her we'll go to Monte Carlo when I feel better."

Sian, away a second year at Ohio's Antioch College, came home. Normally we couldn't have afforded the luxury of a midwinter trip, but she had not seen her father in months and we all accepted this ostensible "Christmas vacation" visit. She quietly observed the gravity of the illness, showing awareness by the tiny frown that knitted into the space between her brown eyes. Crouched on the hospital corridor steps nursing grief, she'd spring up to go back into the sickroom while I had a cup of coffee or a walk around the block. As her father began to rally she read the newspapers to him or sat with a book in her blue-jeaned lap, ready with a damp cloth or a sip of water. When she cried it was alone, softly, in bed; when I kissed her good night the pillow was wet.

Each of us was strong those days in separate ways, protectively held by love and a growing sense of disaster—yet unspoken, still not officially pronounced. I used my daily dose of hope like a drinker sipping a rationed ounce of Scotch: the day Ed said he longed for baking-powder biscuits and ate two of the homemade beauties Harris Russell produced overnight; the afternoon when around the hospital bed we played out the games in Peter Buckman's book *Playground*, the four of us relaxed and laughing as if we were spending a late Sunday morning at home; the first walk Ed took down the hallway, joking with the accompanying nurse about his shuffle; the morning I parked the car a block from the clinic and met Ed out buying a newspaper at the corner kiosk—we walked back to his room planning his trip to Peking before the official United States presidential visit there. Ed was under contract to cover this on his own, not as a member of the presidential press corps. He had never been used by Washington; he wouldn't have wanted to be now. A letter on White House stationery, from Richard Nixon, was sent to Ed as he lay dying, a few weeks before the President was due in Peking to meet with Premier Chou En-lai and, presumably, with Chairman Mao Tse-tung. The Nixon message concerned Ed's health and included a salutation to Ed's "long and distinguished career." It was bitter wine. Relations between the People's Republic of China and the United States were long overdue; Ed was aware of the significance of the presidential voyage, but that did not mean he would now blot out the President's personal and ardent contributions to the twenty years of cold-war hysteria and the tragedy that lay behind those wasted years. Ed's career paralleled the President's only in that they were contemporary, not aligned. We didn't answer the letter and we didn't hear again.

Christmas time came on. Joan decorated a miniature tree which we plugged in on the far side of the hospital room, saving our presents for a postponed celebration at home before the New Year. There was more to come, more work, time to heal and time to—what, we didn't know. Neither how much nor how long.

Friends sustained us all through. Han Suyin and her husband, Vincent Ruthnaswami, sped to Eysins. Suyin, world-wise and world-beautiful (for she incorporates East and West), brought me her practiced doctor's discernment. Her admiration for Ed had grown from years past —as had his for her. Vincent, whose gentleness and perceptivity contrast the strength of his physique—"like a handsome genie from Aladdin's lamp," Ed once said— underscored this attention. With ever so much sensitivity, he and Suyin prepared me for the inevitable I so longed not to face; they helped build bridges to a future in which they knew I had to confront aloneness and finality. Through what made up the remainder of Ed's life they were never out of immediate touch, nor have they been to this day. They are truly "many-splendored."

Chris's and Sian's friends came to the hospital at different days and times, released from work and study: Christiane, like a vibrant, beautiful pony, burst out of the elevator bearing a Christmas-red poinsettia plant and worry in her lovely eyes, Philippe came with roses, Conan and John with steady smiles and a book from their parents. Ed had engendered more than respect in our children's comrades—he was a friend—and though he was too ill to receive them, they were not about to leave him unattended. They came and stayed, for little whiles, outside his door.

The Jarricos were in Switzerland too, Yvette for a medical checkup in a small hospital between us and the lake. Paul picked me up to bring her a plant and get a hug, then drove me on to the other clinic. They knew things were bad but they didn't pry. Paul is warm and discreet and a mountain of strength. He had seen Ed a few weeks before the operation and together they had discussed the China book in progress, as before that they had discussed Paul's film scripts. These two writers were not only friends, they keenly appreciated each other's talent and integrity, leaned on each other's political and literary insight.

Big Paul, one hand on the wheel, mine in his other, drove slowly up the road to Lausanne where snow-splashed Alps blend even higher into misty sky and the lake stretches glasslike under dim white sun. France lay blurry across the water, the Swiss shore close, outlined by homes and hotels and the black sticks of vineyards that on a winter's day look like ink marks in a sketch book. In summer it's all emerald-green and blue.

"Tell that guy of yours the book is great just as it is. Tell him to put a title on it and send it off. He can write more later on—this is right for *now*. Tell him *I* say so."

"Okay, Pauli, I trust you . . . so does Ed."

He dropped me at the hospital entrance. "Tell him . . . tell him we'll have a party when he gets home."

We didn't. There was never again a party time for Ed.

The late-December night before he left the hospital Ed inscribed and gave a copy of one of his books to the surgeon. In it he wrote: "To the man who saved my life—like my body, this book is old and somewhat obsolete, but perhaps there is still some value in each." I watched the doctor's face as he read the inscription; he had not saved the man's life (no one could have) and he had not realized the man thought his life had been saved. I lowered my eyes as the doctor bade farewell. I did not see him again, though he sent a note after Ed died.

We were given a packet of pills, painkillers and sedatives, to be used sparingly: don't overdo! Ed's liver, the body's filter, was so far gone that a "normal" amount of drugs risked creating a hepatic coma. I had no idea of the forthcoming nights when the whole packet could not have stopped the pain or induced sleep. The advice of a professional dietician was: let him eat whatever he wants. This tight-faced man indicated, in sum: the man's dying; if he wants something particular to eat, let him try it, eat as best he can; there is nothing else to be done.

There was much else to be done; we found this out later. The only thing we got from the dietician was a bill for his "service."

Nudging our way through cotton-white fog on the iciest night of the year, I drove Ed home. The plate-glass hospital doors had swung shut; with their closing, surgeons and specialists became shadow people to be contacted at office hours through remote secretaries or recorded messages. Our neighborhood doctors took over, in touch with the original team, but that was of little meaning at three o'clock in the morning when the day's pills were finished and interminable hours stretched ahead before the next prescribed allotment. That was the time of aloneness for us both, caught in hurt and fatigue, heightened by my inability to overcome sleep and stay awake with Ed. Undone by my illness, I'd drowse in the chill hours before dawn, leaving him huddled on the couch dealing with his pain. Why is the nighttime so *awe*-full—low point of resistance, physical and emotional, pierced by phantom fears? Though ours had become real enough; we had to push them away, beat them aside.

Daytime was better. Light reduced the night terror, brought a semblance of normality, allowed us energy to move around our broken health. Dr. Panchaud came by every day unfailingly, mornings or afternoons. His robust frame made Ed look even frailer, but his strength was stimulating. The two men talked together as they had for years, only now conversation was low-keyed with Robert's deep rumble supporting Ed's slower speech. When a pallid January sun became enticing, I'd walk to the village and back with Ed, an obvious strain for him, this outing, but a need nevertheless, a pinning of himself to normal activity. He had always walked to the village.

"I'm weak!" he'd say almost in surprise as he stumbled in spite of snail's pace and my sustaining arm. "It's a slow recuperation."

"Let's go just to the corner field."

"No, to the village." He insisted, I went along. His thinness made him look taller, his height increased by a long camel's-hair coat and the Chinese fox-fur hat he used against the cold. Our village neighbors watched from a distance; they had no idea how to help.

An evening came when Ed felt well enough to dine downstairs. Chris and Sian opted for a rare night out, seeing us first comfortable in the living room, with music and cocktails in front of the fire. Ed sat in the "new" chair —one I had admired in a Geneva store window with him and he'd gone back to buy for my birthday in July. It's striped in Scandinavian orange and rust against a wheaten white; the colors match the room, alive with books in the wall-wide shelves Ed had carefully measured, cut, placed and polished. He wore his Christmas pajamas and robe, I a long wool skirt. The decorated tree was still up (an unusual one with two stems; after acquiring a house and garden we began to buy Christmas trees with roots encased in a tub of earth. This was our third, and the children planted it in the garden after the holidays, Ed choosing the spot). Light flickered from the candles on the coffee table between us; we talked about our books, the children, the leak in the roof, while Joan Baez's silver voice filled in the pauses. I see us there each time I enter the room, now that it's all past, because at that moment, then, in isolated ease, it seemed the way it had always been—until Ed shook his head "no" to dessert, looking suddenly shattered, and I helped him up to bed. He could hardly crawl in. That night promised to be rough; there was only one permitted pill left until morning.

I once played the part of Emily Webb in *Our Town*. That night I remembered the line when she returns after death to watch her family busy, self-absorbed at home, and she cries, "It goes so fast, they don't have time to *look* at one another." It was true. Threatened with separation, we clutched at moments that ordinarily would have been taken for granted; like falling stars they crossed our darkness, leaving a strange sense of reality—time went too slowly or too fast in the face of death.

When Ed felt like it we worked together upstairs in the "petit salon," the white-walled, dark-beamed study adjoining our bedroom. There a wood fire blazed and tea was on the ready. Ed dug into files and continued doggedly with his book, encouraging me to go ahead on mine. I dragged along distractedly. Yet bits of talk and work echoed those happier days after our return from China, when we had anticipated the publication of both books together, my first attempt and his mature analysis. By the fire glow those winter afternoons we experienced a coming together again, a reuniting as if the splitting of sickness had been an aberration, an ugly distortion, and actuality was far removed from pain and fear. It was transitory; disaster waited.

Telephoning Branson O'Casey, who had worked closely with him on his 1966 film of China, *One Fourth of Humanity*, Ed said, "I'm not getting any better and I need to finish some work." Branson is a composite of uncommon joy and uncommon sense; we are deeply intermingled. She flew immediately from her home in London; she stayed to type dictated letters, put film business in order, give of her brightness, mixing in leftover hours with Joan and me, the three of us in search of answers to unanswerables—a puzzling one being how we had returned full circle to conditions that had led Ed to the hospital in the first place; the specialists had performed, withdrawn—and the pain was back and bad. Our incompetence seemed insurmountable as we watched Ed in his battle for time, insistent on recovery, at least for a little while. Most of the work during this period was done with a recorder; Ed's faltering, fuzzy voice lies captured in those metal discs along with Branse's warm energy expressed in that combination of speech and love so particularly hers—the British accent spiced with the native North Carolina tang. It was Branse who, the day she left, accompanied Ed on his walk to the village; we didn't know it would be the last one he'd take.

Meanwhile, Joan's home in Arnex became a wayside hostel, with doors wide open. Branson stayed there, my sister when she came; often there were two or three overnight guests. It was a center for special messages and mail, where I went to thrash over increasing problems, and sometimes, to release an accumulated ache of worry, the better to face Ed again with momentary calm. I could cry aloud there, bathe my face and go home to talk more easily with Ed. Joan relayed news to anxious friends, and brought us the gifts and delicacies they left with her rather than risk disturbing us. The Russells' supply was steady: Ursula's homemade jams and pickles in accompaniment to Harris' cornbread and biscuits—their way of sending support.

I had stopped the door delivery of mail by this time; too many people were writing messages of foreboding and fear. I did not want Ed to see these, nor speculations on his illness in the press. Either the children or I went to the post office; we screened the newspapers and letters before bringing them upstairs to Ed and reading them aloud when he wanted to listen. He enjoyed familial accounts and was avid to keep up with world events.

Joan's phone and address were used for replies from those who were searching out medical help in other places. Ed's brother and sister, ready-packed but hesitant through my hesitancy to suddenly appear as if death were imminent, kept in constant touch by mail and phone. Mary, in New York, was combing the city for advice, Branson and friends in London were doing the same. The replies were similar: Switzerland has everything known to medical science in the treatment of cancer, the same drugs, techniques, skills and highly qualified specialists; nothing would be gained by changing locale. The medical report,

74

which had been agonizingly slow to materialize after the operation, had finally been forwarded across land and sea, and in response the serious, controlled voices of doctor friends admitted it was bad, very bad. What they and others had to give was generous personal attention, concern for my health and the children's well-being. Dying is expensive in our society; the financial costs loomed paramount: "Can you handle it? Do you need money? Let us help." We were profoundly touched. I especially remember the look on Ed's face when he read a letter from an old friend who he knew could not easily afford the offer of his savings whenever we needed.

All this was large comfort but I sought the miracle that would make Ed well. The reply from China didn't promise cure, but it offered concrete physical help and that was a near miracle to me. George Hatem wrote urging us to consider a trip to Peking, where every attention would be paid, every comfort administered, every bit of scientific knowledge applied. His letter was immediately followed by one from Premier Chou En-lai, along with supportive messages from Chairman Mao, his wife, Chiang Ching, and the Premier's wife, Teng Ying-chao. This communication of friendship and acknowledgment had brightened a dreary morning for Ed in bed. Too weak for effort that day, he had listened as I read the contents aloud. Ed made an unusual remark for him, revealing a kind of surprised recognition of such attention. "I must be the only American who has had a letter like that from Premier Chou!"

He dictated a reply:

Dear Friend,

I am still overwhelmed by the warmth and generosity of your sympathy and the concrete proposals to help in my present predicament made by Chairman Mao Tse-tung, Madame Chiang Ching, yourself and Madame Teng Ying-chao. That you should pay attention to such a detail in your extremely crowded lives and even send your envoy, our friends Ambassador and Madame Chen, in person with your greetings and invitation is extraordinarily moving and at the same time, humbling. I have not replied concerning your proposal to come to China for treatment or convalescence because my immediate situation incapacitates me to plan such an action. I am still very weak. I am in the midst of a series of chemotherapy treatments and tests which now cannot be interrupted for some weeks, after which there might be results and a break when a transfer could be feasible. I am sending details to Dr. Ma Hai-teh, and shall let him know our future plans as soon as possible. The kindness you offer attracts my wife and myself very much, but naturally requires some planning and also depends on my recovery of minimal mobility. It is of course greatly disappointing not to be in China now but perhaps I can be more useful later.

Permit me here to add my condolences to those of the nation in mourning the recent loss of a man great in his revolutionary services to China, Chen Yi.

With full reciprocation for the deeply appreciated sentiments expressed by Chairman Mao, Chiang Ching, Teng Ying-chao and yourself, and strong hopes for the successful outcome of the forthcoming Sino-American meeting and other brilliant China initiatives, and may good health continue to guard you.

Sincerely,

Edgar Snow

Soong Ching-ling, widow of China's revolutionary leader

Sun Yat-sen, had also written. Distressed by our illnesses she sent a letter offering her personal help. Soong Ching-ling had long been Ed's close friend; she became mine during our visits to her home in Peking. In that special place in her heart for Ed she included his family. It had been touching to see the photographs of Christopher and Sian in her home—we had sent those pictures to China from the States when the children were about eight and six. Ed had a deep admiration for this heroic woman whose values had placed her, at the cost of family ties and wealth, on the side of the revolution, steadfast and spirited. Courageous all her life, she gave me courage in her message from across the miles.

For Ed, too, it meant courage—to have the strength of China offered to him, a foreigner. But the courage reinforced his determination to recover that "minimal mobility," to finish his book to the extent that he could leave his vast notes and diaries, and then go to China, upright if possible, to devote himself to convalescence.

I was not optimistic, but faced with his will I could not cut off his hope. I turned to my sister Kashin, in California. Kashin is tall and thin and sweet and strong. She knows what struggle is, for she has had her share, and she knows how to share in struggle, for she has overcome. She answered at once that she was preparing to leave for Eysins.

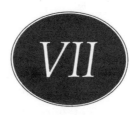

In some respects Geneva is the center of the world. Its compact airport daily dispenses, with an efficiency perhaps unequaled for its busy-ness, a crisscross multitude of travelers; during our years there we have never felt out of touch. People constantly pass through, on business, on pleasure, or on the way to somewhere else. It's one of the blessings of this cosmopolitan capital and one reason why our residency grew Topsy-fashion—we never caught up with all the people here to see.

Ruth and Hans Maeder, so close to us we chose them to be unofficial godparents to Chris and Sian (disliking the idea of "official" ones, but "in case we both disappear") come over twice or thrice a year. We rarely saw them as often or as intimately when we lived in New Jersey, and they at their Stockbridge School in Massachusetts. Our friendships go back to pre–World War II, though not jointly until much later, after Ed and I had married and discovered that he had known Hans as an anti-Nazi refugee in the Philippines, that I had known Ruth as a theatrical literary agent in New York and that somewhere during intervening years they had met, married and built their lives around their school. It had been our intention to send Chris and Sian there to be educated, but our years abroad turned into many and the children grew up Swiss instead of Stockbridge.

Over on a quickly planned trip, the Maeders telephoned as a matter of course. Catching the quiver in my throat, they drove by to take me out to talk. Hans felt something should be done immediately, and though Ed was seeing no one but his family, Hans was firm about a short visit to determine possibilities that whirled through his active mind. I brought him unannounced to Ed the following morning and the two men spent time alone upstairs beside the fire in the "petit salon." That day in January marked the entrance of the Chinese into our shattered lives. When Hans came down from his talk with Ed, I showed him the special-delivery letter which had just arrived. Peking had acted: Mao Tse-tung and Chou En-lai were sending a medical team of doctors and nurses. They wanted to escort us all back to China. Relief flooded Hans's face.

"That's good, they'll save him if anyone can," he said in his direct way. "You must take him to Peking."

"I'm afraid Ed won't go," I replied. "He wants to stay here, where he has all his notes and material. He's determined to finish his book."

"Make him see it won't do any good if he stays here and dies," said Hans sensibly.

I knew the decision was Ed's. I knew, too, by now,

that the help the Chinese were offering was more than anything the rest of the world could offer—for his book, and for what was left of his life.

Sparing Ed an official visit, Chen Chih-fan, Ambassador from the People's Republic of China to Switzerland, discreetly invited me to the Chinese consulate in Geneva. We had talked there before, Ambassador Chen, his wife, Wang Ching, and I, while Ed was still hospitalized in Lausanne. On that occasion, knowing the medical report was on its way to Peking, knowing that Ed lacked the energy to face anyone in his immediate postoperative state, and assuming that the ambassador would feel it necessary to pay a courtesy visit, I had parried Chen Chih-fan's probing about the seriousness of the illness. Tactfully he had let me do so. Now I was asked once again to visit with him and his wife.

Leaving Chris and Sian with Ed, I went to Geneva and was received in the consulate drawing room—that special mixture of formality and casualness that characterizes the reception rooms of all the Chinese government's homes away from home I have seen: heavy tables and chairs geometrically arranged, antimacassars that slip out of place, cloisonné ashtrays and tins of Panda and Chung Hua cigarettes, a huge mounted copy of a Mao Tse-tung poem in his original calligraphy, and the Chairman's portrait counterbalanced by an exquisite old-style embroidery of the postrevolution Nanking Bridge over the Yangtze River.

Dressed in pants and jackets, the Chens served tea and Wang Ching held my hand as I wrenched out the true horror of Ed's illness. Their sympathetic understanding made me realize I need not have withheld the truth from them at the beginning. Consoled, I listened to their words from Peking. A medical team, assembled in China, was at that moment in Pakistan boarding a plane to take them on to Switzerland. I learned that the Swiss authorities were waiving regular formalities and would in cooperation issue visas to the Chinese immediately on arrival at the airport. A Peking hospital suite was being prepared to accommodate all four of the family—Christopher and Sian could be with their father as well—and an Air France plane would be set up with a bed in a private area for a direct trip over. Above all, I was told to pay attention to my own health and not worry any more; everything possible was being done.

George Hatem was included among the Chinese en route to Eysins. Hatem, an American-born doctor with a Swiss-earned medical degree received in Geneva, now a citizen of the People's Republic, had been Ed's friend since the early thirties when the two young men had slipped through Kuomintang war barriers to undertake the hazardous trek to distant Pao-an in the northwestern badlands, where the Chinese Communists ended the Long March. That adventure resulted in Ed's writing *Red Star Over China* and in Dr. Hatem's remaining with the revolutionaries as a much-needed medical man. "His arrival," Ed wryly noted, "doubled the Western-trained medical force" of the Eighth Route Army.* In Yenan he met and married Chou Su-fei, a beautiful young movie actress who had gone north to join the ranks of the revolutionaries.

* See the chapter entitled "Doctor Horse" in *Red China Today: The Other Side of the River.*

After Liberation, the Hatems returned to Peking, where they still live, near to their daughter, son and three grandchildren, all of whom inherited the remarkable Hatem eyebrows. Ed and I had spent memorable times in the lovely home behind the gray brick wall that separates their compound from a lakeside drive in Peking—hours of talk under the grape arbor, with Su-fei presiding over waffles topped with honey gathered from the Western Hills, or Dr. Hatem producing the crazy concoctions he lumped under the general title of "dry martini" after he found that to be my preferred cocktail. I could not have hoped for more consolation than the reunion of these two once-upon-a-time-young pioneers. (Later, when I saw Chou En-lai and his wife after Ed's death, Teng Ying-chao replied to my thanks for their help by saying, "It was a natural thing for us to send our doctors when you needed them; after all, Ed brought us a doctor when we badly needed one.")

As we waited for the medical team, chemotherapy treatments, begun at the local hospital, continued. Ed wanted them, pinned his hopes on them, though professional opinion indicated small chance of success or remission. So much depended on unknown factors, we were told; some terribly ill people had gained months, some years, some no time at all. It is harsh treatment; Ed's sessions were three times a week, each more than four hours long, and were particularly distressing because the pain in Ed's back, alleviated only temporarily after surgery, made lying supine and motionless excruciating. Chris, Sian and I took turns sitting by the cot reading aloud, watching that he didn't move and dislodge the needle strapped into his arm vein. Once it jerked out; painful probing was necessary to remove any traces of poison injected into his body. I wondered if the pain was worth it, or if a different method of administering the chemicals couldn't be used. There seemed to be no alternative.

After each session we brought Ed back home hunched in the station wagon. He wanted no more hospital confinement; that was apparent. On a visit when Joan was the chauffeur he said, making a face at her, "Thanks a lot. Remind me sometime that I owe *you* a trip to the hospital." He had six chemotherapy treatments in the weeks before the Chinese arrived and he seemed worse than ever. His feet became so swollen that I couldn't lace his shoes; his thinness was terrifying. Some relief came in warm water; helping him in and out of the tub several times a day and sometimes at night, I was appalled at the steady, shocking loss of weight. Deliberately standing in front of the mirror, I'd stretch out the big bath towel to shield him from the image. But he brought in Sian's little American scales and watched his weight go down. It was Joan who took it upon herself to fight the weight loss; she whipped malt and eggs into milk shakes, cooked fresh lobster, sought out ripe melons to accompany prosciutto—anything to tempt his appetite—and added up calories as earnestly as a novice investor counts fading assets during a stock-market crisis. Others had ideas that sparked momentary expectation: special diets, special clinics, special cures. People were so urgent, we so in need, that sometimes a wild hope blazed.

Ed knew little of this fruitless search. He was fighting his own battle, not often acknowledging the approach of death. Only once, in nighttime anguish, he moaned, "I never expected this to happen so early in my life," a reversal of a remark he had made before the operation: "I've lived so long I've come to think of myself as indestructible." Another time, on a sullen, rainy afternoon (is it better to die in the springtime or at full summer bloom, or would such natural radiance make it harder?), we talked about belief in God. We had both been baptized Catholics, had both long ago left the Church, but Ed never carried the fear and superstition instilled in me from convent childhood and dark confessionals (Heaven, the flames of Hell and Purgatory, somewhere off in chilly space a shadowy void called Limbo, and God a mixture of omnipotence: Chief of Police, J. Edgar Hoover, Franklin Delano Roosevelt—and virtue: St. Francis of Assisi, Jude the Impossible, to whom I prayed when things were all up with me, and Santa Claus). Ed's focus was mankind and his belief was in a continuancy of matter and spirit, all becoming part of the universe. He kept a wooden card file with a constantly growing collection of quotations (Mao Tse-tung, Shakespeare, Mark Twain, Lewis Carroll, Clarence Darrow among many others, including both Marxes, Karl and Groucho). A quote from Albert Einstein—"That deeply emotional conviction of the presence of a superior reasoning power, which is revealed in the incomprehensible universe, forms my idea of God"—is tagged in parenthesis by Ed: "(mine too)." For the title of his autobiography Ed had used, from the *Chuang-tzu*: "To know that Heaven and Earth are but as a tare-seed, and that the tip of the hair is a mountain: this is the expression of relativity . . . Beginning and end are like a circle. Growth and decay are the succession of transformations. Where there is end there is the beginning." He had been intrigued

84

by Mao Tse-tung's remark to him, during a conversation in 1965, about the eventuality of "going to see God." I think both men agreed there was *something,* but neither was pushing to find out by going.

For several years we had known and come quietly close to a practicing parish priest in Geneva. This had begun through a Vietnam "study group" of which he had been an instigator and in which we had been participants. Modern in his views, casual in his dress, firm in his faith, he represented the best of two worlds: religious precepts freed from the distortions of bias and cant, and international brotherhood which includes all mankind. When I asked him if he should talk to Ed (my convent legacy still churns beneath carefully accumulated layers of emancipation), his reply was simple and decent: "If he wants to talk to me, he'll ask and I'll be there right away. Don't force anything on him he doesn't want. He has nothing to worry about with anybody—including God." If he had taught my fifth-grade catechism class, I might still be with the Church.

We left it that way, and our conscientious man of religion came by from time to time to sit in kitchen warmth and talk over a cup of tea. Occasionally I'd go upstairs to say casually that he was there, but Ed was occupied with trying to live and that was that. (I think Ed's name got mentioned quite a bit those days when our friend was saying mass.)

For Ed, the inability to sleep was even harder to endure than the increasing pain. Prescribed sedatives were no longer effective, if they ever had been. For a few days we supplemented them with calcium (my idea gleaned from Adelle Davis)—calcium pills, calcium powder, calcium in warm milk—but it proved to no avail. The one night I succumbed to early deep sleep, Ed, unaware of what he was doing besides seeking relief, took three or more pills in a short space of time, thrashed about the dark house, slipped on the stairs and jolted to the bottom. Chris heard the crash, jumped out of bed, helped his father back upstairs and remained with him until morning. It frightened us all terribly; the children and I agreed to night watches divided among the three of us.

So we clung together, in malfunction—we had so much at our disposal that I couldn't grasp why—until the Chinese came, literally out of the sky. Our neighbor Ursula Russell called their coming "instant history." While we waited for them, Kashin arrived. Ed got up from the day bed to kiss her when she came upstairs. It was an effort of love—on both parts.

We talked in whispers that night, Kash and I, while Ed dozed. "How . . . does he look to you?" Steadily, with so little solace to offer, Kash replied, "He still looks like Ed in his eyes."

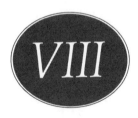

VIII

The Chinese were expected in the early afternoon on January 24. Sian and Chris had finished washing lunch dishes and gone up to sit beside Ed. I was downstairs waiting in the kitchen, which, receptive to visitors by its big window, faces the front of the house. We have a main entrance door on the courtyard too, but most people head for the kitchen, where we like to gather more often than in the large living room. It's an old farm kitchen, dark-beamed, tile-floored, and we left it basically as it had been except for some newer plumbing, checked cotton curtains, a copper hood capping the stove, and a red-painted, built-in wall cupboard. (I had planned the color otherwise, but we happened to find a leftover can of red paint in the house and little by little things became covered with that bright hue. It was traumatic enough for me when Ed painted some carefully scraped ceiling beams crimson, but the day he trimmed dead branches from the pear tree and sealed the saw scars with red paint—the tree looked as if it had developed a case of the measles—I put my foot down. Luckily, it was the end of the can.)

It's a big room with a bright (red) desk and an Ed-made wall shelf. He loved to do carpentry and was always relaxed with a saw or hammer in hand. This has led in other homes to linen closets, mantelpieces, fish pools, and a long time ago, a complete remodeling of my old dollhouse for Sian. When we moved to Eysins, one of Ed's pet projects was fastening a couple of Tang horses (ceramic copies) to the chimney tops on the slippery tile roof; he intended these as identification for the name he chose for our house —"Deux Chevaux." One horse agreed to stick in the cement base, the other refused and eventually a windstorm wrecked the first. Out of Tang horses, Ed dropped the idea of naming the house and it is simply called by the postal number, but the kitchen shelf Ed built remains staunchly fixed to the wall and contains a heap of books, the best splattered being *The Joy of Cooking* and Julia Child. There are also several years' worth of *Gourmet* magazines, tattered dictionaries, guidebooks, road maps, sheet music for Sian's guitar, paperbacks, and a sprinkling of Mark Twain and Mao Tse-tung. On one wall is a Douglas Gorsline still life of a French honey pot, and above the mail-cluttered desk and phone is the ink sketch of our house that Joan made for a Christmas present the year we moved in. The door opening to the courtyard entry is covered with newspaper clippings and notices: WAR IS NOT HEALTHY FOR CHILDREN AND OTHER LIVING THINGS (*Another Mother For Peace*); RESIST, Daniel Berrigan's LETTER FROM THE UNDERGROUND (clipped from

the *International Herald Tribune*); and emergency telephone numbers: *Feu* (it's a volunteer fire department);
Hôpital; Plombier (which is Monsieur Rosat roaring over
on a motor bike when pipes burst or the washing machine
gets stuck).

Waiting for the Chinese there, in that room so full of us
and our family ways, I prepared for tea, puttered with the
avocado plants, fidgeted—my mind flickering back to the
doctors and nurses we had met in China, the visits Ed and
I had made to village clinics, to city hospitals. I remembered the time I saw Ed cry in a Peking hospital ward
where we talked to a man who, months before, had suf-
fered third-degree burns over most of his body. He had
insisted on getting up to show us that he could walk, and
he read aloud from Mao Tse-tung with the little sight left
in his remaining eye. His face was a total scar; later he'd
have plastic surgery to make it easier for people to look at
him. A transport worker, he told us he wanted to live, to
use what remained of his body in service to others, to continue the great change in his country. His ward mates
listened understandingly and the young doctor remade the
man's bed before he got back in. I was moved, naturally,
but I almost broke up when I saw tears on Ed's cheeks. The
burned man had touched something deep down.

Another vivid memory was in a hospital ward for women
with malignant tumors of the uterus caused by wild cells
which, instead of resulting in pregnancy, form cancerous
growths. Fifteen patients, in various stages of age and illness, all childless, were going through treatment in an in-
credibly brave effort to retain lives and fertility. Most of
them would already have been cured by the early removal

of the diseased uterus, but all of them wanted to bear a child. I entered the room with dread; I left with a feeling close to elation. Fatality was being combated with science supportive of the women's courage and their confidence in the doctors and nurses, all of whom stressed the need for the patients' belief in cure and their participation. Discussion sessions, Mao Tse-tung classes, are held each day in the ward; staff and patients study and talk together. Mao teaches that the history of mankind is from the realm of the impossible to the realm of the possible. About half the women, we later learned, whose wombs were cured of choriocarcinoma have produced babies. The attention to that human need, in a country where population control is stressed, was impressive.

Of course this occurs in other places, other societies; devoted doctors and nurses are not exclusive to the Chinese, nor is there in this world a scarcity of patients determined and encouraged to conquer severe illness. Distinctive to me was the depth and extent to which the doctor-patient-people relationship—a mutual guidance and communication—was applied. Part of the unexpected in China with its mass of people was the attention I saw paid to individuals (and the attention these individuals pay to China). In medicine, emphasis is placed on the person who is ill, ahead of the illness. While everything possible is done to treat the disease, personal circumstances are of primary concern. We had seen this, Ed and I, in many hospitals, big, medium, small—some so small and bare that they seemed to be makeshift. Regardless of equipment, surroundings, size of staff, the commitment was there. The English scientist Dr. Joseph Needham calls it a "humanization process." * Han Suyin speaks of the "*human* factor—resolution, will, conscious mobility." † It surmounts an obvious lack of technical equipment in many places by the ampleness of attention paid to human beings and the preciousness with which life is regarded, as in the admonition to all medical workers that they *not* treat the patient as a disease, that the person comes first. This I knew.

Still, for *us*—how would this be applied to *us*? I puzzled. Would it be overwhelming—would *our* kind of freedom be curtailed? My feelings were mixed; I knew Ed's were too, despite the immensity of the response. Though I was frantic for help, I was not eager to be "dominated." Nor was Ed. It was one reason why he did not want to return to a hospital—anywhere.

I was deep in thought when three black limousines splashed slowly through the driveway puddles and George Hatem climbed out of one car, walked in the rain through the kitchen door, put two arms around my shoulders and hugged me to his big chest. "Su-fei sends love," he said.

"Shag" (as I had learned to call him from Ed) was there smiling, with grief in his soft brown eyes. I closed my own and felt skyborne with relief.

Then the grave Chinese: Dr. Huang Kwo-jun, tall, kind surgeon from Peking, with English his second language; Dr. Chang Chen-kuen, dedicated eyes behind glasses, cancer specialist from Wuhan; Li Chung-ping (Little Ling), round and petite—Shag called her "Dumpling"—an experienced nurse in the care of the very ill; Chang

---

* In speech published in *China Now,* journal of the Society for Anglo-Chinese Understanding, February 1973.

† *The Morning Deluge* (Boston: Little, Brown, 1972).

Yi-fang, a big-boned, strong-faced woman with doctor's degrees in both Western and Chinese medicine; tender Pu Shui-lien, head nurse of a Wuhan children's hospital; and Ting Shu-ching, acupuncturist and anesthesiologist, who at thirty looks like a schoolgirl with a smile that makes her face as sprightly as her name. I bit back tears to shake hands. A familiar form stood in the doorway, Hsu Erh-wei —short-cropped hair framing her sensitive face—our guide, interpreter and companion through all the miles of China when Ed and I had traveled together a year before. We clung to each other for a long moment. Ambassador Chen and his wife filled the entry hall; beyond them, through the open door, Li Pen-kan and Chao Yin-chuan, comrade chauffeurs, beamed as if they had created the scene. From that point on, through all that was to come, I was never alone or afraid.

I don't recall how we got settled, who went where, except that Shag immediately went upstairs. He sat on the bed, holding Ed's hand, and I left them together; it seemed right for them to be alone. Chris and Sian were the ones who thought of taking tea to the chauffeurs waiting in the cars.

"Imagine *us* making tea for the Chinese!" They giggled out of nervousness. "They probably won't be able to drink it."

"Do they take sugar?"

"*Mais non!* . . . But they'll probably need it—it's *tea bag!*"

They took the tray out in the drizzle, a first shy overture to the strangers in their home. By late afternoon it was as if we had known each other for days and by sundown as if we had known each other for years, so easily did they slip into place. That night, when I saw Ed relaxed and at ease, I slept straight through for the first time in weeks.

Earlier, after the bustle of welcome died down, Shag had stood fixed before the portrait of Ed that hangs in the "petit salon." It is the only one ever painted of Ed, and the creator is special to us as both friend and artist. Douglas Gorsline's brush is guided by a camera eye for detail and a sensitivity that instills content with perceptive dimensions of movement, life and depth, whether in a Côte d'Or wheat-field scene, a waterfront in Cannes, or the face of a guitarist off the streets of Pigalle. The portrait reveals Ed in five faces, painted on different occasions (that is, when he could be caught) over the length of one year, blended into composition and form. It was done during a period of abstention from smoking (like Mark Twain, whom Ed read for pleasure and sustenance, he found giving it up easy—he had done it often); the unlit cigarette dangles from his fingers as he, cross-legged in baggy gray pants, reads, thinks, converses. He and Branson, who was visiting with us at the Gorslines' home in France, had talked together for the better part of a morning while Douglas captured the beginning of Ed on canvas. "I'll *fascinate* him," Branse said joyfully to Douglas in a promise to hold Ed still.

We had spent many happy, relaxed weekends and longer at the Gorslines' farm outside Dijon, working in the vegetable garden, concocting semi-Chinese and in-depth French cuisine, exploring the countryside, where on several occasions we came close to unrealistically acquiring property under the spell of a French real estate agent who, taking our Walter Mitty excursions in earnest, almost made deals with us for several wrecked *châteaux* and dilapidated *manoirs*. He gave up in dismay the day we prowled over a hill-perched village farm whose stone-tumbled dwellings magically appeared rehabilitated and decorated in our eyes until we counted up the cost. Marie Gorsline and I, two Mrs. Blandings with dream houses in our heads, were scrambling through the interior darkness of the main building, guided by the polite French gentleman, when a bat suddenly swooped over our heads. We both grabbed Monsieur with wild shrieks, and he promptly dashed out of the house in panic. After recovery in the sunlight he bade us definite, if shaky, adieu, and that was the end of the house hunting. From then on we contented ourselves with trips back and forth between the two practical and habitable homes we already had; Douglas finished Ed's portrait during several of these visits and hung it, himself, by a rusty wire suspended from the stone wall in our upstairs sitting room. There Shag came upon it and said, "Whoever painted that knows and loves Ed deeply."

"He's downstairs," I told him. "Come and say hello."

Marie and Douglas had recently driven from France and were lodged at a nearby hotel. Like everyone, they had felt a huge weight lift when they learned the medical team was en route to Eysins; they were staying on to help prepare for the trip to Peking if that was to be. They had stopped by almost as soon as the Chinese had arrived. Seeing the cars in front and the crowd in the kitchen, they had unobtrusively entered by the other door to build up a fire in the living room before slipping away to leave us alone. Later Marie told me of her alarm when smoke started pouring out of the fireplace after she and Douglas got a blaze going. They discovered that the draft was closed; she was frantically trying to clear the air by pushing the terrace door back and forth when Ambassador Chen entered from the hallway with the newcomers.

"The ambassador thought I was trying to keep the door from blowing open—he pushed while I pulled, and I explained, for some reason in French, what I was doing while he tried to find out in Chinese what I was *doing!*"

Eventually they understood each other, Douglas got the hot damper open and the Chinese shook hands with the sooty couple. It was the beginning of friendship, founded on Ed, and it was to lead to Marie and Douglas fulfilling a long-held wish, a trip to the People's Republic of China to paint its people and its land. Douglas became the first American to record on canvas the strength and beauty of China after the Cultural Revolution.

They came as friends as well as experts, these Chinese citizens; they came with undivided commitment. They saw at once the inroads of the dreadful disease and they knew the trip to Peking was no longer feasible. The evening after they arrived Shag said, "We had made a home out of a hospital for you in Peking; now we'll stay here and make a hospital out of your home." And this they did, with expertise, patience and devotion, making it possible for their American friend to spend his last weeks with his family in relative peace and calm. Without them this would not have been achieved, and a return to routinized hospitalization would have been inevitable. Through them, home and hospital blended; with the personal—the *person*—put foremost, Ed was no longer a "case." They were able not only to release him from the worst of his physical misery but to bring him a tranquillity, a dignity in dying that made it more bearable—not only for him but for me, for our two children, and for our families and friends. They were to affect everyone they met.

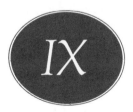

IX

Shag Hatem stayed with us at Eysins, occupying the small
library at the back of the house where light filtered in
through the winter-bare fruit orchard beyond our garden.
Soon his room turned into a miniature pharmacy, the book-
shelves cleared to accommodate a jumble of jars, bottles,
liquids and pills—Chinese calligraphy mixed with Latin
inscriptions. (The beams Ed had painted red seemed right,
then, with the new use of the little den.) Once in a while
Dr. Panchaud and the Chinese team worked back there
among the medicines—Shag's fluency in French and Chinese the means of communication.

Housed at the Chinese consulate in the suburbs of
Geneva, the doctors and nurses were driven back and forth,
day shift replacing night shift. They were in coordinated
attendance twenty-four hours a day. No agonizing period
had to be endured while a helpless nurse, dependent on an
absent doctor or supervisor to change instructions, held

back an urgently needed analgesic until a precisely scheduled hour. It was a hitherto inconceivable care, managed with a harmony that forestalled any feeling of disruption in our normally casual household—beyond the pervading, oncoming death, whose inevitability was now a part of us. We knew there wasn't much time and we used each day fully, strengthened by professional presence, grateful for informality and the respect for, the tolerance of, tension—for we grit our teeth in the face of death under the best of circumstances. The relief from physical pain was not always total, but it was enough to make hours bearable when they would have been excruciating.

Another relief was the integrated relationship between the Chinese (I include Shag Hatem with them, as he is now a citizen of the People's Republic) and our family; between the Chinese and Swiss doctors; and between the Chinese and all the varied people they encountered in our home.

Among these was Madame Nolfo, the young Italian woman who comes twice weekly to help with chores. It is she who irons our never-ending laundry, who attacks dust and cobwebs, makes windows gleam again after splattering rains, performs miracles with potted plants, sews on buttons and replaces broken zippers. Born into a big Sicilian family twenty-seven years ago, she knows when a storm is brewing while the sun still shines, why the hens aren't laying a normal supply of eggs, and how to cook a fabulous rabbit stew with Italian herbs from her garden. She and her husband have two children—Salvatore, age nine, a bright slim lad in the village primary school, and Rosetta, who at four accompanies her mother to work, follows her from room to room, crayons on innumerable scraps of paper, or when days are balmy, creates flower-cities in the graveled garden paths. Madame's French is more rapid than mine, more colloquial, and strongly flavored with Italian, which is the language she more easily reads and writes.

If she had had the education she wanted, she would have become a seamstress; as it is, she saved up for a sewing machine and Rosetta is the best-dressed child in the village. It didn't take Madame long to understand, without being told, the gravity of Monsieur Snow's illness (her reaction was more vigorous polishing and a steady supply of fresh eggs), and it was shortly after she met the Chinese that she decided they were very special people. I doubt if she had seen a Chinese up close before; I can tell from the look in her black eyes when someone isn't up to snuff, and her eyes revealed that she thought *they* were. Occasionally, not liking guests we have had in the house, she has retreated into herself, and that has been that until the end of the visit—though she is never impolite.

When Rosetta developed a sore throat, Madame brought her directly to Dr. Chang Chen-kuen. She would have gone to any of the Chinese, but the first she encountered that morning just happened to be Dr. Chang, who was sorting sheets in the laundry room behind the kitchen. He tended the little girl with consideration, and Rosetta's stiffness softened under his attention. Madame soon managed to acquire several creaks and aches and proudly accepted a proffered tin of Chinese Tiger Balme. (Joan's tennis elbow got the same treatment.) And later, after the weeks together ended in death, and the Chinese were returning home, Madame dressed her son, her daughter and herself in Sunday go-to-meeting clothes, went into the living room, where we were all saying good-bye, and with dignified formality led her children around to individually thank each of the doctors and nurses, the interpreters, the drivers, and the ambassador and his wife. *"Ils ne sont pas comme les autres,"* she told me. *"Les Chinois sont tellement gentils."*

It became the word for them. *Gentil* can mean much more than "nice"; with a certain inflection it becomes a crystallization of fineness. Dr. Panchaud remarked, *"Comme ils sont gentils!"* when he first met them. Soon after, impressed by their work methods, he added, *"Et comme ils sont habiles!"* Our neighbors the Grangers said the same. I slipped over to them once in a while to apologize for the coming and going of cars in front of their house. (They didn't mind at all—at that time a good part of their world was what went on outside the kitchen window. Since then they have acquired a television set, but from the time we moved next door, the Grangers have taken in stride a parade of visitors *"chez les Snow,"* rock-and-roll at two in the morning and motor bikes roaring off in the midst of their afternoon naps.) When I assured them of the care being given to my husband, tears would slide down Madame Granger's face. *"Pauvre Monsieur Snow! Ce n'est pas juste,"* she'd cry. Monsieur Granger would nod in accord. *"Mais ils sont magnifiques, les Chinois. Ils sont gentils."*

They were even more than that; they were efficient, tireless, and above all, available. There is yet a limit to technology; there is none to humanity, beyond our own making.

Any fear that our privacy would be upset soon disappeared; as the Chinese brought control we had more privacy, more opportunity to be together, Ed and I, the children and their father. Without planning, we gave each other time alone with him, private time which often meant just holding hands, being still, and close. It was a blessing.

Another was the discussion sessions that began the day after the Chinese arrived. Whenever we felt like it or whenever it was deemed important, Sian, Chris and I joined the group that gathered between each change of outgoing and incoming shifts. Robert Panchaud was frequently there, as was Kashin (who spent all day and evening with us and retired at night to sleep at Joan's home down the road). Twice or three times a week, and nearly every day toward the last, Ambassador Chen Chih-fan and Wang Ching were in attendance, leaving pressing duties behind at the embassy in Bern to become supportive, unobtrusive representatives of their country in our home. Hsu Erh-wei arrived each morning to interpret, an art she combines with warmth and skill; in her spare time she worked on a translation of the long list of Chinese opera terms I needed in English for my book. The consulate chauffeurs, waiting to drive into Geneva, would sit in on some of these meetings, listening solemnly, following the reports with concern and interest; they were part of the whole.

Together, the doctors and nurses would study and explain charts in front of us, exchange ideas, analyze problems and suggest possible methods of better, more effective treatment. There appeared to be no hierarchy and no division; Little Ling, her round face pink with earnestness, was listened to with as much consideration as were the eminent surgeons. If any of us, the family, didn't understand something, it would be explained. I don't mean that a detailed medical analysis was given every time a question was asked, but practical answers were available as we needed or wanted them: how the edema (that frightening swelling in Ed's feet) was being lessened, why changes were made in the intravenous drip mixture, and what went into the carefully composed diet, for of course, the Chinese said, diet was of enormous importance, requiring professional supervision and scientific control. I was not to fully realize until they explained that pain is caused not only by severed tissues and nerves striving to heal in the postoperative period, but also by hunger and thirst, and it can be placated through properly administered nourishment of an ill-functioning body. The Chinese had the time as well as the desire to explain not only the causes of pain but what they were doing to lessen that pain in their patient. For Ed, it was of immense benefit to have his failing body get fed.

It was a strange dietetic arrangement, but food got, and stayed, down, a little at a time in bites and nibbles. Meals were not precise or routine; there was no fixed schedule. "Better to eat a little when wanted; keep something appetizing on hand," said Shag. Along with carefully measured amounts of phosphorus, vitamins (K was important), glucose, cortisone, digestive medicines and Chinese herbs, there was a range of favorites, the foods that had always tempted Ed's appetite and that he could still enjoy: bits of smoked salmon, Swiss chocolate, Chinese soups, puddings, poached fish, eggnogs, and Joan's homemade ice cream, spoonfuls of which Ed was able to eat and enjoy long after he couldn't manage other foods. When Joan had gone through chocolate and coffee, and strawberry made with fruit plucked and frozen from her garden, she asked which Ed preferred. His answer, like a kid's, was "Butter pecan." Joan got out every cookbook we had, found no recipe for it, and made up her own delicious concoction. Pecans cost a fortune in Europe and are not easy to find. She found them, and Ed, with help from everybody, ate up the can of ice cream. Joan promptly made some more.

The daily exchanges took place in our living room; it had gradually gained a noticeable similarity to the reception room at the Chinese consulate: tables and chairs (with the exception of some frankly weathered wicker porch variety, ours are mostly Chinese) lined up face to face in two precise rows; teacups appeared next to the Chung Hua cigarettes, the tea tins and the ubiquitous Chinese thermos bottles with their unlimited supply of steaming hot water. We already had a picture of the Chairman on the wall, a Chinese poster made from a photograph Ed had taken in Pao-an in 1936, of the young Mao wearing Ed's eight-point Red Army cap on his long black locks.

Discussions took place in Chinese, and Hsu Erh-wei or Shag interpreted. Dr. Huang's English was excellent, but he generally used Chinese when his comrades were present. Sometimes his rare, gay laughter mingled with Ed's upstairs, set off by Ed's trying to make a pun in Chinese. The doctor's tact and tranquillity generated ease and was of particular meaning to us; we no longer had to hold back questions or be "patient." There was no feeling of secretiveness or estrangement. A community had formed and we were an integral part, no longer outsiders waiting in an impersonal corridor for piecemeal information, hesitant to intrude in an area beyond our ken. It was as simple as that. We shared questions, answers, knowledge, limitations, large and small, good and bad; the sharing brought us together with the man upstairs and did much to make the inevitable easier to accept.

Our meetings were microcosms of what I had seen and read about Chinese society, where combined study and analysis are practiced at all levels. Everyone, in whatever activity or work, discusses problems and progress, successes and failures, in group sessions that call for full participation, with self-criticism as a requisite, and political analysis (Marxism-Leninism–Mao Tse-tung Thought) as the guide. William Hinton, who has spent many years in China, writes that Chinese socialism "involves the radical transformation of every kind of human relationship, of human motivation, of human consciousness; it involves the release of the enthusiasm, the energy, and the creativity of the masses and the development to the fullest of the capacity of each individual." *

Dr. Joseph Needham, in a speech in London in 1972, delivered the following pithy impressions of study sessions he had encountered in China:

> Now I don't have to talk about all the obvious things like total social security, or medical aid and medical services, or education or transport or about all these hundred and one necessary things. We can take it as read, because we all know that these things are well organized in Chinese socialist society. But I would like to harp a bit on the question of human values. Take the

* *Turning Point in China* (New York: Monthly Review Press, 1972).

slogan which was very important during the Cultural Revolution, especially during the fight against the rightists' policies, about "putting politics in command." Again I don't repeat this exactly as it is, for I translate: "putting human values in command," because this is really what it means. And what this implies is many things: for instance, not putting "economic laws," nor bureaucratic authority, nor high technology, nor yet high cultural attainment, nor even perhaps perfect efficiency in running things in command. It means putting human values in the place where they belong, and getting people to understand each other, to work together and to be at one with each other in a way they have never been able to be before in human history. And when I say "perfect efficiency in running things," of course there are arguments in various ways about this. It may be that a very much larger amount of time is spent in China on meetings of committees and councils, but in the end this may be a more efficient way of running things than any kind of dogmatic or imposed disciplinary authority. And here I have in mind what I think of as "College Councils," because the Chinese are always meeting in groups in just this sort of way. You find it everywhere: in every factory, every shop, on the workshop floor, at every railway station, in every college and university, every hotel. It always amuses me in Chinese hotels to see the staff disappearing into rooms every now and then all together, and then coming out an hour or so later having had a good talk about their problems. Why did something go wrong on such and such an occasion? Why didn't they treat that tiresome foreigner with greater patience and get him that unusual drink he wanted so much? It would be better perhaps to do such and such a thing another time in another way, so in future they would be better prepared. A thousand detailed problems come up in running an hotel, and they don't have it all dictated by somebody in the office. It isn't a question of "them and us" —them in the office handing out instructions. It is deciding for ourselves. This works through every stage and level of Chinese society from the bottom to the top.*

In the area of medicine this stressing of human values results in an understanding not only among the staff members and the administration but between them and their patients and the patients' families. I am told that this often extends to other patients who, when able, become active in the care of their fellow invalids. Personal difficulties are discussed together—anxieties, finances, children, marital upsets, housing, etc. Nothing is overlooked in the effort to work together in a supportive relationship whereby fear, ignorance, mistakes, nonparticipation or selfishness is brought out in mutual investigation and mutually decided action.

What I had heard and was now witnessing in my husband's care is borne out by the experience of others. Dr. Hatem has told me of such practices in the Peking hospital where he is employed, the Fu Chin Men Wai. Leigh Kagan has reported specifically on a psychiatric hospital in Tientsin which she visited in 1972. She describes the use of the study method and of Mao Tse-tung's writings in hospital application:

> . . . Bewilderment over the use of Mao Tse-tung Thought in the treatment of mental illness may be natural as a first reaction. We may think of Mao as a political thinker, organizer, strategist, dealing with questions of power on a grand scale. But his philosophical and epistemological writings are designed to enable

* *China Now*, published by the Society for Anglo-Chinese Understanding in February 1973.

people to organize their perceptions and formulate a materialistic view of reality. Only if we refuse to grant that Mao's writings are meant to construct an approach to reality can we dismiss their use in the treatment of mental illness. And after all, patients when cured return to the society in which they live and work.

. . . the hospital itself operates on the premise of maximized relations between patients and the entire medical and hospital staff, *as in hospitals throughout China* [italics mine].*

During a visit to China in the autumn of 1972, an Australian woman found herself unexpectedly hospitalized in Peking. Later she wrote of her experience:

> Since my return, people . . . have said, "What a pity to visit China and spend your time in hospital." I can only say that this time gave me an insight into China life and the organization of Chinese society which I could have gained in no other way. . . . in the quiet room of that hospital I experienced something so enriching and enlightening that I could only be grateful for this opportunity to think and learn . . . There was none of the isolation which we associate with illness. One felt the warmth of human concern, not thrust upon one, but constant, kind and every-ready to be called upon. One retained one's identity, for one was an active member of the team. . . . it was an amazing experience. Doctors helped nurses make beds, nurses helped orderlies with domestic work. Everything was discussed with the patient. There was none of the furtive conspiracy of hidden charts, information kept back, secret discussions which, to us, seem essential attributes of hospital treatment. Doctor

* "Report from a Visit to the Tientsin Psychiatric Hospital, March 1972," in *China Notes*, Vol. X, No. 4 (Fall 1972), published by the East Asia Office of the National Council of Churches, 475 Riverside Drive, New York, N.Y. 10027.

conferred with doctor and doctor with nurses in the presence of the patient whose help was needed in working the cure. Never did I hear a brusque or impatient voice or see anything but a cheerful and solicitous face. One could express one's thanks but the answer was always the same: "Don't thank us, it is our duty and we can do nothing without the co-operation of the patient." How can a patient fail to be co-operative, for co-operation was based on understanding, and confidence was induced by the sight of the professional members of the team working together in harmony and equality.*

These are personal insights, fragments of a huge scene, as was our experience, but it was in these ways that needless suffering was overcome, endless complications eliminated. The writers experienced, as we did, care that was complete. It was inestimable assurance, this confidence that nothing would be left undone or overlooked in unceasing effort to make Ed more comfortable and us, his family, more at ease. We knew this would last to the final moment.

*"In a Chinese Hospital," by E. M. Christiansen. *Eastern Horizon Magazine*, Vol. XII, No. 1 (1973).

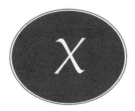

I carried a subconscious worry that broke through as Ed
grew weaker: efforts might be made to prolong his life at
the cost of additional suffering. When I brought this out,
I was assured it was not to be; the essential was to alleviate
pain, to soothe tension and emotional stress, to ease—not
prolong, when there was no hope—the physical process
of dying. Though I wanted him as long as possible, I did
not want him one minute more than was decent for him
to live.

We both needed to be together, but it took one bad moment for me to learn how important it was to Ed that I
stay close. The presence of the Chinese allowed me rest.
Still convalescent, I slipped into afternoon naps, and to re-
lieve the strain I talked with friends who stopped by. An
evening came when, after several hours' absence, I went
upstairs to find a forlorn Ed who cried out, "Where have

you *been!*" From that instant I tried not to be out of reach for any appreciable time.

When he asked for me in the night, one of the Chinese would call me from the room across the hall to which I had moved, and I'd sit by the bed, sometimes to read aloud until sleep came to him again. He slept more often as the Chinese administered sedatives that by-passed or were not too harsh on the ruined liver. This lessened the danger of poison, and since the composition was periodically changed to avoid habituation, they continued to be relatively effective. But Ed had been an irregular sleeper in the best of health, and had always relied on books to fill in the cracks of night. I, with a need of eight or nine hours of complete unconsciousness, had envied him the shelf-fuls consumed in those "wee hours" when he'd read practically anything that found its way to, or under, his bedside table: mysteries, encyclopedias, the Bible, a biology textbook or a French grammar, science fiction, and a pile of magazines and papers we were always going to "clear up" and hardly ever did. Stand-bys were a worn copy of *Alice in Wonderland*, G. B. Shaw, and Mark Twain: *Huck Finn* is as well thumbed as *The Mysterious Stranger*, and the one-volume Shaw is penciled with notes. Ed was a scribbler, even in borrowed books.

A hospital bed had been brought in to replace the big one Ed and I had shared. It was jarring to me, this mechanical metal substitute, but for a sick person it was far more practical and comfortable with its overhanging hand bar and a crank-up elevating mattress; it also gave increased space and facility of movement in our small bedroom. Christiane's Christmas poinsettia, a reminder of the same blossoms that had seemed to me like red stars on the front steps and doorway of the Peking Hotel the year before, sat on the window sill; beyond, the fields stretched down to the lake, and Monsieur Granger could be seen as ever, puttering among his winter cabbage. I got out pastel sheets, a gay bedspread; the yellow-flowered back-rest cushion Mary Heathcote had sent from New York livened the room, and the soft-colored pants and jackets the Chinese wore on top of their bright pullovers bore no hint of hospital uniform.

Shag dressed Western style, usually in slacks and sweater. On a rare visit to Geneva one evening, he donned the sports jacket he had worn on arrival in Switzerland. It was eye-catching, a thick, handsome, multicolored tweed, different from any I'd seen in China.

"Where in the world did you *get* that, Shag?" I teased.

"From Chou En-lai," Shag replied seriously. "When I saw him the day before we left Peking, he asked me what I was going to wear in Europe. I had on my nice old padded jacket and I said, 'This—this is what I'm going to wear.'

" 'You are *not!*' said the Premier. 'You'll disgrace us all in that.' He called a tailor and I had this the next morning."

Shag turned around for inspection. A black beret, perched on his head, added French zest to the general effect. "I feel sort of odd in it," he admitted shyly. "I liked my old jacket . . . but I guess Chou En-lai knows more about what's being worn in Europe than I do."

Chou En-lai has many facets; I would not have placed haberdashery among them until Shag gave credit to the Premier for his jacket—if Ed and I had not had a similar experience in Peking. We had met with Premier Chou a few days before going to Shenyang, the capital city of China's northeastern province of Liaoning. He told us it would be cold up there that time of year and cautioned us to dress accordingly.

"Wear warm coats," he said.

"We're fine," Ed assured him. "We've borrowed sweaters and ski jackets galore."

The Premier shook his head. "Coats," he repeated, "you need long coats."

Ed mentioned that he had never seen the Premier himself in a coat. It is well known that he had for years gone hatless and coatless even in midwinter.

"I wear a coat now," said Chou, ". . . if I *have* to."

The next day two tailors called on us at the hotel, laden with swatches, patterns and tape measures. They came from Chou En-lai and we were having coats. We set off for Liaoning in a couple of "his" and "hers" in dark-blue wool, hip-length, mine half-belted in the back—a purely ornamental addition to break up the straight line but a puzzlement to the tailor, who nevertheless put it on.

When we next visited the Premier, we wore our coats. "You were right," we thanked him, "we needed these."

"They're too short" was his comment.

We called them our "Chou coats" and wore them steadily in Switzerland, where winter months seem as cold to me as China's northeast did on my one visit there, but maybe that they're a gift from Premier Chou warmed our blood. Kashin must feel the same, because she borrows mine. My sister, used to California, shivers in Swiss winters like a kitten left out in the snow and is never far from any available source of heat. To ensure a supply of firewood, she

joined Chris and the comrade chauffeurs in splitting logs
and got to swinging an ax like a pro. We called this her
lao deng—Chinese for "manual labor."

Indeed, the house ran as smoothly as a commune brigade. Meals appeared for the Chinese as if by magic.
Actually, they were brought each morning and evening
with the shift of nursing teams: big canisters filled with a
variety of delicious foods prepared by the kitchen staff of
the consulate. Accompanying hot rice was made in our
kitchen by one of the on-duty Chinese, who gladly demonstrated, when any of us stood by to watch, how the grains
were cooked. Nurse Ting seemed to be chief "rice chef,"
but I couldn't tell the difference between her technique
and Dr. Chang Chen-kuen's, though his slow-paced English helped me verbally through the process. (I still use
American rice, but that may not be cricket.) Eventually
we began experimenting with soy sauce, pickled vegetables, Chinese vinegar, and wine. The Chinese invited
us to eat their food and we in turn offered them our Western specialties, including oatmeal cookies, nut brownies
and pizzas. I think we liked their cuisine better than they
liked ours; however, we are overfond of Chinese cooking
—I had gained twelve pounds in my five months' visit to
China. I didn't lose any of them on the delicacies brought
to us from the embassy and consulate, but I did find out,
when we had too much, that a "chao tze" retains its sub-
stance in a deep-freeze as crisply as a saltine cracker.

It was Shag who relished the cooking he hadn't had in
years. It was fun to watch him down a pizza on which
Chris had heaped a mound of golden Gruyère, or Madame
Granger's apple tart, or a breakfast of pancakes, bacon

and eggs. Would his "Chou coat" button in the front? we wondered. But Shag was not deterred; he is a gourmet in several languages.

The kitchen became the focal place, where we gathered to whisper, wonder, sometimes to laugh or cry, sometimes to work. Kash spent time at the kitchen desk answering telephone calls, taking messages; often she had to disconnect the phone to help take care of shopping, answering mail, driving into town. There were things she could do which the Chinese couldn't, and one, important to me, was acting like a normal sister under these abnormal conditions. Her natural sense of fun remained and she shared it generously, drawing us into badly needed play, even being silly when the occasion arose, like hopping about with Chris on the crutches Mary had left behind, both of them giggling as they chased each other outside in the courtyard. It was good to hear laughter; Ed heard it too and he'd wink at the sounds of Kash being "funny" with the kids. Twists of humor wound in and out of those days. The sharable moments we brought to Ed, others were incidents blown up disproportionately, amusing only to those they happened to, but that was the way it was—tension relieved by a droll mistake, sorrow forgotten in seconds of fun. We dangled on the verge of laughter or tears, the latter somehow easier to control, perhaps because they had been part of us for so many weeks.

Kashin, aware of a lack of coat hangers in the front entry but preoccupied with priority obligations, had kept that need in the back of her mind, and once when the Chinese chauffeurs entered the kitchen as she was preparing lunch, she interpreted their gesticulations toward the second floor as a search for coat hangers. Knowing where there were plenty downstairs, she nodded emphatically and ushered the two men into the big closet off the kitchen, pleased with herself at this comprehension. They admired the hangers, nodded as she nodded, smiled as she smiled, remained puzzledly in the closet when she left them to their choice—then came out to point up the stairs again. They had a message for one of the doctors and he was on the second floor —it had nothing to do with coat hangers. We roared together when Kashin told me this, tears pouring down our cheeks as if it were the funniest thing that had ever happened. Another incident, this one because of our efforts to keep the press at a distance, set off peals of laughter. The Chinese sought no publicity and we were completely occupied, without time or desire for interviews or statements. Reporters kept phoning and finally came calling at the house. Kash got accustomed to handling them with her usual grace, but the first encounter proved she had a lot to learn. Answering a knock at the door (we have a cowbell instead of a buzzer and it seldom gets "rung"), she faced a young man who asked if the house was the Snows' residence.

Kash hesitated for some time and then answered, "I don't know . . . I'm not sure."

"But," said the reporter, "don't you know where you are?"

Kash remained adamant. "No," she replied after a pause, "no, I don't."

The man was at a loss to continue. Bowing as if in vague agreement, he retreated to his car and drove off.

There was, too, an overall unrealness in daily events

where normality was undercut by what was happening to the central figure in our lives, the one who, slipping away as the days passed, was being cared for by foreigners in our midst quietly determined to "turn sorrow into strength," as they put it. Though they became our friends, closer than some of longer duration because of the intimacy that bound us, they remained specially Chinese. I remember how this struck me over and over in their physical behavior: Pu Shui-lien's strong young hands washing Ed's face as if they were handling fine porcelain; Ting Shu-ching's deft fingers massaging his brow, injecting needles or extracting blood with delicate precision. Always the gentleness and the smile.

The torture of lying still during hours of intravenous drip was done away with by the simple expedient of a mobile needle inserted in a hand vein and taped in place, leaving Ed free to turn at will, to move his arms. Remembering the hospital chemotherapy sessions when movement had practically been restricted to breathing (and I had wondered why), I was surprised by this tiny apparatus. "It's a needle we use on babies," they explained. "Babies can't be strapped down." When Ed wanted to pace a bit or go to the bathroom, tall Drs. Chang or Huang took turns holding the apparatus up high, following Ed around "like the old emperors with their umbrellas," they said, laughing. Ed laughed too. It was an odd sight.

Nails were put into ceiling beams in the "petit salon" so that the drip attachment could be hung from spots above the day bed or over the couch where Ed liked to be when he felt like sitting up. I watched the Chinese fix one of these nails; the scene was like a photo from Chinese theatre, a combination of traditional Peking opera gesture and model revolutionary content—title: "Nurses and Doctors Serve the People." Chang Yi-fang and Pu Shui-lien were directing Chang Chen-kuen's placement of the nail; he, dressed in a black cotton jacket, poised to strike when the women agreed on the right spot, waited motionless on top of the ladder, his face raised ceilingward while they below held their arms outstretched in support and direction, arrested as in the prints of theatre wood-block illustrations I had seen in innumerable Chinese magazines. I almost expected them to be in stage make-up.

"There, right there," said the nurses. Dr. Chang struck a single blow, the theatrical effect disappeared as he descended the ladder and the three turned to greet me standing in the doorway—human beings, not Peking opera characters. But oh, so Chinese!

The considerate tread of cotton-shoed feet, the ever-ready smile, the suppleness of hands, the simplicity, the clarity of behavior, the serenity of these men and women marked them with a quality that would seem almost monastic if one didn't know it to be quite the opposite—a revolutionary attitude toward life, a different kind of ethic. If I were asked to be more specific, I could only say that with all that was done, they restored balance to our shaken lives through conduct that reflects values on a high level of human behavior.

Because of the usable combinations of English-French-Chinese we had developed, Hsu Erh-wei's services became less needed than in Peking, where experienced interpreters were in demand for the forthcoming visit of U.S. officials and press. Little Ling accompanied Erh-wei back home.

Two Chinese nurses were flown over from Algeria, where the Chinese were participating in the construction of a countryside hospital and in the education and training of Algerian medical personnel.

Erh-wei and I said good-bye to each other across the space of twin beds in what had been the guest room before I moved out of where Ed and I had intended to sleep for years. We were shatteringly aware that whenever we met again it would be without Ed. The three of us had become fond of one another on our trips across China; that affection had been shared by another interpreter-companion, Yao Wei, to whom I now sent, in Erh-wei's care, the soft, strong leather gloves Ed had barely had time to break in. Yao Wei, I knew, would wear them with regard for the man who had been his teacher and friend.

Afterward, downstairs, Little Ling, face atremble, returned my embrace and accepted the Swiss music box Sian brought from her room as a present for Ling's small daughter back in Peking. Christiane, part of our family since she and our children attended Swiss school together, had appeared that day with an armful of peach-pink roses, her normal gaiety subdued. We all stood together in front of the fireplace while she took our picture. It turned out sepia-colored, but it's full of warmth.

The embassy car drove the two young women off to the airport and returned that evening with the new nurses, Wu Bao-hsien and Li Tze-yin, who had spent days and nights traveling from the Algerian countryside to our home. Slight and pretty, they were also thoroughly tired, but they didn't let on for a second.

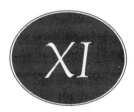

Shag hardly ever left the house; he was the last of us to go
to bed, the first of us up in the morning. In his easy way
he was available to everyone, yet always ready in a corner
of the room whenever Ed wanted to talk, to turn, to get out
of bed. He was up past midnight urging me to get some
sleep; he'd given Ed breakfast before I awoke. He was constant and so was his strength and wit. It was clear what a
perfect companion he had made those far-ago days when he
had gone with Ed in search of the "Red bandits" in China's
forbidding northwest.

Word spread that George Hatem had come with the
Chinese doctors; he would have been deluged by callers if
he had responded to all the telephoned messages. He answered a few from old friends of Geneva days and finally,
after special pleading, he agreed to talk at an evening meeting with the medical personnel of the local hospital. From
what Sian and Chris reported that night, he could have

gone on through the next day. I did not attend and regret not seeing him, with his round girth enclosed in the bright tweed jacket, the center of a fascinated audience absorbed in the formation of Cultural Revolutionary Chinese medicine. There couldn't have been a "barefoot doctor" within three thousand miles, but maybe potential ones sprouted that night. Though Shag is not a proselytizer, he is a dedicated worker who knows more about present-day Chinese medical practice than almost anyone else in the world, and his behavior bears witness to the good possibilities of man.

As with them all. How they come back—vignettes of the Chinese comrades: Erh-wei curled up in the Scandinavian chair in a rare moment of rest, her pretty nose in a copy of Jane Austen; the tireless chauffeurs chopping wood, making tea; Wang Ching carrying out dishes or wielding a broom like the good mother she is, embassy protocol put aside in the face of illness; Chang Yi-fang trying out her school French: *"J'ai deux enfants comme vous, c'est bien, c'est bien"*; she'd repeat it occasionally for comfort, reaching beyond our language barrier, and as everything she did was *"bien,"* we got along wonderfully well. Her compassion was like an embrace whenever we spoke or passed each other; I felt she would have cut off her hand to stop the death in our midst. Her dark eyes shone more darkly when she looked at Sian and Chris, alert to their loss. (Sian's name is special to the Chinese—*an* means "peace" in their language, and though the whole word, *Si-an,* translates literally into "Western peace," we had said as we named her, if there is true peace in the West, there must also be peace in the North and the South and the East.)

And scholarly, quiet Chang Chen-kuen—a Peking-opera buff. I should have guessed he'd prefer chess. In his red wool sweater and his precise, measured English, he took time to explain details of the new revolutionary opera, knowing my interest—he steeped in Chinese theatre, I an amateur by contrast. Ed wanted us to talk by his bed; when he dozed off I'd tiptoe into the next room to make notes or add a little of Dr. Chang's wisdom to my book.

There was sparkly-eyed Comrade Ting, who transliterated Lois into "Lo-ee-su" and called Kashin "Mei-mei" (Younger Sister), and who waved an energetic *hen hao shu shi* ("good rest") as the car carried them off each evening. Kashin and I would stand in the circle of light cast from the open kitchen door to wave back until the red tail-lights disappeared down the road, then we'd shut ourselves off from the outside cold to welcome the newly arrived shift.

I recall Sian, long brown hair tumbled over bent shoulders, reading softly to the gaunt figure in bed, her hand caressing the limp one on the blanket; Chris carefully shaving his father's pallid, stubbly cheek with Shag's electric razor (a present Ed had taken him on a visit to China); Dr. Panchaud's great hand smoothing Ed's forehead, his strong features fragile as he faced the approach of death and his inability to stop it.

We were all-participant. Farewells took place almost without our awareness; continuing contact cushioned the break. There was no more waste of time or energy, no more puzzlement, no chaotic grappling. Ed saw that and appreciated it.

Marya Mannes has written about "the ever-increasing

fight of the individual to maintain and exercise his rights over matters affecting his life and death, his mind and body." We knew that those rights had at last been restored by the Chinese easing Ed "truthfully but gently into death." * Reduced to dependent weakness, he escaped humiliation and was able to use the strength that remained with decency. He knew, as I did, how this had become possible.

And what of Sian and Chris? We shared a great deal, but there were things we could not share; to talk of them then might have opened floodgates too painful. It was their first intimate experience with death. They were losing the father whom they adored, and their loss was an early one that denied a future for the mature relationship that they would have had with him in later adulthood. They had been through the hospital scene and the strained confusion at home afterward. They knew the difference the Chinese had made; no one could have been in contact with them for five minutes without becoming sensible to their principled behavior. Through them we had acquired focus. Our energies could be applied, without dissipation, to adjusting to rupture with a sense of perspective, an insight that comes at such a heightened time. Mourning mingled with understanding, grief was lightened in distribution, both weights borne by all of us. It was the Chinese who made this happen, but it was the young people who summoned restraints that further protected us. In knowing what to share and what not to, what to continue and what to give up, they grew into maturity without obvious

* *Last Rights* (New York: Morrow, 1973).

change. They had their special friends over as they had had before, played everything from the Beatles to Bach on the stereo (Ed groaned over Dylan, but then, he always had, with a twinkle—it was a family joke), and they kept their private problems (interrupted commitments to school and work) outside the immediate threat, maintaining a pattern of normality, a control, while extra readiness, casual but constant availability, discretion, edged the new responsibility they took on. Their choice of behavior, conscious or not, was fine.

Of course, the presence of the Chinese among us was extraordinary. Since neither of our children had been to China then, they had no personal way of measuring to what extent those few people reflected their society in general. This came to them, a lot, through Shag Hatem. Their father had written that "not Marx but life experience had made an emotional radical out of Dr. Hatem before he reached China." * An emotional radical is not that unusual; what is unique about Dr. Hatem is China. His more than usual desire to be of service to mankind found terra firma in a social base that nourished and guided him when young. Through the practiced man, with his informal American speech, Christopher and Sian gained a better sense of the *why* of the Chinese in our home.

Then, in the last week of Ed's life, Huang Hua arrived en route from Addis Ababa to New York City, where he is China's permanent representative to the United Nations. Detoured by friendship and the skeins of history, he brought a message from Mao Tse-tung to the dying Amer-

---

* *Red China Today: The Other Side of the River.*

ican for whom as a student, thirty-seven years before, he had interpreted the night-long conversations with the young Chairman Mao in his loess mountain cave in Pao-an. Shag went upstairs with Ambassador Huang, and the two men who had shared that time with Ed stood silently at the foot of his bed, laughing with him when he roused himself to say in surprised recognition, "Well, we three old bandits."

Huang Hua took two days out of his demanding schedule to stay with us, to talk to our son and daughter as if they were his own, to confer over medical reports, to talk with Dr. Panchaud, to assure us of all help possible from the People's Republic. One late afternoon the rumpled ambassador, his jacket unbuttoned, sat on the stone hearth in the living room, a bowl of Joan's ice cream in hand, and talked to Chris and Sian about the Chinese people's appreciation of their father's contribution to a world understanding of the Chinese revolution, about their esteem for his honesty and integrity. As dusk closed in he and Shag reminisced about the years spent with Mao Tse-tung and Chou En-lai, about battles and ping-pong games and the life of revolutionaries in the Shensi mountains. Shag told how Li Na, Mao's baby daughter, had played with Shag's cigarette lighter and got burned. "It's all right," said her father. "She has to learn sometime."

There was a break in Huang Hua's voice as he delivered a message sent to me by his wife, Ho Li-liang. Ed and I had spent most of our five months in China with them in 1970; we had expected more meetings in a future that now would not include Ed. Did Ed think of that when Huang Hua said good-bye to him? I think he was too tired. Huang Hua looked gray and sad.

In retrospect, individual pieces of the mosaic shine clear; the whole is misty. Some seconds seemed forever, days passed too fast, nights were sectioned by awakenings, dreams and sleep. I clung to good moments—when Ed laughed, when he responded warmly to my kiss, to the sound of music from downstairs, when he listened attentively to a news report on the radio; I endured the bad— a groan, a grimace of pain, the terrible yellow of his skin, the beauty of his head when in profile the skeletal thinness wasn't apparent and he looked pathetically young in the lamplight and I couldn't bear the vigorous, vital man I had lived with being cut down so soon. Though I was certain that if he had had a choice, to live a long, horizon-bound life that culminated in senility or to have had the full one he was leaving before he was ready, he would have chosen the latter. I understood that and could smile later when I read the protocol to the will he left behind, disposing of his "brief loan of assets here." I could see him as he wrote it, elbows on his big desk (a wooden door placed on two filing cabinets), fingers twisting, twisting that front lock of hair, his grin breaking out as he added at the end of the cold legal language: " . . . certain personal requests to be carried out in consultation with Lois, of course, whom I hope to meet later—if she can arrange it!"

I don't believe I could have borne being left alone with him ill, unable to help him, or to have him back in the impersonalness of a hospital. Balance came through the Chinese. I could therefore help where I might have cringed, cry in release where I might have raged in despair. I think I am basically a strong person. Certainly I am an emotional one. I know now why I almost cracked during the period of Ed's hospitalization, and why I was able later to bear unbearable sights, like Ed taking that long trip from bed to bathroom—a distance of two yards—slowly, carefully, with infinite attention, raising his foot mountain-high to proudly pass over half an inch of door sill, determined to be in control and not wet his bed. The Chinese understood; together we helped him gauge his way, together we helped him back to bed. It was such a little thing and it meant so much.

Such attention *is* given in our hospitals; I have had it myself in a comfortable and moderately priced clinic in Geneva. But it is rarely constant or consistent or freely given, except by uncommon modern Florence Nightingales. Again and again I thought of our special position, not to mention having the care in our *home*. In Europe, hospitalization is still relatively inexpensive, though costs are rising. England has socialized medicine; France has a decent, extensive health-insurance system; in Switzerland more citizens are adequately covered than not. In the United States the cost of serious illness, the cost of dying, can mean financial ruin.* For the poor it can mean hell; it is the wealthy who come off best and even with them the quality of care is largely up to individuals who may

* The *New York Times* (July 6, 1974) put the average cost of patient care in New York City's voluntary hospitals at "A staggering $150-a-day level," with an additional augmentation in price cited for the immediate future. In Switzerland, too, costs are going up; today a private room in an average hospital costs approximately $45 a day.

126

or may not be able (or willing) to give all that is required. In China medical costs are practically nothing and everyone is covered. The state takes care of financial needs, companionship is built into communal life, sickness is tended to within the communes, and in the cities by medical workers reaching into every neighborhood and by street committees organized block by block to shop, cook, clean and even entertain. Nobody has to worry about unpaid health insurance or uncollectable social security—nor the reliableness of care. This is not charity. It is a conscious, considered political act by a government clearly opposed to neglect, to waste, and led by a man who long ago stated "of all things in the world, people are the most precious."

I can think of only one thing comparable in our society —the widespread and sustaining help, the *community,* offered to millions by Alcoholics Anonymous. AA's diversified membership works in an ensemble of unity, mutual care and attention, with a true spirit of service from and by those who know its worth. Through them, barriers are broken, people are aided at any hour, time and patience are expended freely and fully.

Our own razed barriers did not mean trespass on private areas. I went to the garden when I needed, to walk up and down with the wind in my face, despondently protesting the fast-dwindling time, and conversely, in the motionless night, I stood alone by dark windows half hoping Ed would slip away in sleep and the pain wouldn't be there any more for him. I railed at myself, apart, for thrown-away time, for quarrels, impatience, misunderstandings, selfishness—for moments I'd give the world to undo. But

I could sit by Ed whenever we felt like being alone—a doctor or a nurse always at hand, reading or studying in a nearby room, but never interfering. Once Ed asked me for a Scotch on ice, as if he were trying to test himself or force himself into normality, and I brought it to him and helped him hold it to his lips. He took a sip, sighed "Terrible, it tastes terrible," and we were both cruelly disappointed that it didn't taste the way it should. It was the same with cigarettes; he finally couldn't smoke any more, but he liked my having one myself and he said it smelled good. It was Joan's ice cream that he enjoyed up to the end.

Tender moments were watching Drs. Huang and Hatem, black head close to gray, poring over a medical dictionary of generic terms in a search for European components of Chinese medicines not available in Europe; Wu Bao-hsien's quick smile responding to Ed's mumbled Chinese as she massaged his temples with her supple fingers; Ambassador Chen passing out chocolates from the enormous box that had appeared in the house; he and Madame Chen tiptoing to the sickroom door, gazing in unperceived, and retreating silently to talk to each other downstairs, forming a message to Peking and the concerned friends there; the chauffeurs washing up after tea, murmuring to each other in tinkly sounds and laughingly accepting a frosted cupcake offered by one of us in the kitchen; and the day Ed asked Sian to cut his hair: "Not too short, there's not enough as it is."

"You look like a Beatle, Papa," she teased, clipping carefully as he sat up in a chair with a towel around his neck. I swept up the gray snippets from the floor and, unnoticed, put them in an envelope in my desk drawer.

There was the morning when Ed, sitting up to nibble at soft-boiled egg on toast, felt well enough to say he'd get back to his book the next day—"do some work, it's good for my morale." Comrade Ting nodded approvingly—*"ko yi, ko yi"* ("can do"), she encouraged, while Li Tze-yin clapped her hands in delight. These moments stung with joy.

The book occupied Ed's mind. I was wrung by his need to finish it. He had managed further work on some details and had agreed with the publishers about the inclusion of the 1964 and 1965 articles based on talks with Mao Tse-tung and Chou En-lai, as they had not found print in entirety before in the United States. I would not—could not—pressure him, but when it was finally very late and very dim, and when I *had* to know, I asked him if he wanted his book to be published as it was. He had held out for such a long time. That day he said, reluctantly, "Go ahead."

It was defeat after a good battle, and the battle was more than half won—as Paul Jarrico had said, there was a book, it just wasn't the full one Ed had struggled to complete. He fought incapacitation as only a journalist with a world's scoop and a deadline can fight, conscious of the historical developments of which he had been forecaster and participant. His close friend John Service was to write later:

> . . . He lived through much darkness. But he also saw the day when American policy seems to be turning away from two decades of unrealistic and insensitive ignoring of the human realities in China—and in countries like Vietnam. He lived, too, to see his own great contribution to "mutual friendship and understanding"

being recognized at last on both sides of the gulf that had existed so long. The best possible memorial to Ed Snow will be a continuation of the start that has been made toward the re-establishment of friendly relations with China.

Ed was to have accompanied the President to China* as correspondent for *Life* magazine. The trip itself was a vindication: to have been present seemed fitting as a kind of recompense for the long years in the wilderness. My own first reaction—and I'm sure of many others—was to think: how tragic that Ed could not have gone! But thinking on it, I am not so sure.

Ed would certainly have savored the historical significance (and irony, after all that had happened in the past twenty-three years) of an American President shaking hands with Mao Tse-tung and Chou En-lai. But what could be done with a "correspondent" who was much more than that, who was really a ghost at the banquet? How could he be expected to be one of the horde of confused and frustrated news and television men, watching from afar and gleaning little? He could hardly be a member of the President's party (though that might be fitting). And his presence could only have posed awkward problems for the innate courtesy of his old (and very important) Chinese friends.

I prefer, myself, to remember Ed as we see him in that magnificent picture taken with Mao Tse-tung on Tien-an-men. Surely, in the animated look on his face, we see the flash of fulfillment and the awareness of destiny achieved.†

Lastly, and shining clear, is our friend K. S. Karol, walking into the kitchen to hold me in a bear hug, his face

* Not quite correct: he was to have gone ahead. Once again.

† "Edgar Snow: Some Personal Reminiscences," in *The China Quarterly* (April–June 1972). Ed and John Service first met in 1935 in Peking, where John Service was a Foreign Service officer and language attaché.

creased with sorrow. He had been in Italy, deep at work on his next China book,* telephoning for news until, worried, he took a plane from Rome. His cracky voice was consoling, his presence dear. Much younger than Ed, born in Poland instead of Missouri, experienced in revolution and in war, Karol is a writer of the same integrity as the man he admires. From his first visit to our mountain house in St. Cergue years ago, he has been of importance to all of us. Together he and I went up to look at Ed faded into the pillows. He never knew Karol had come; he had slipped that day into a coma, not to be conscious again.

* *The Second Revolution* (New York: Hill & Wang, 1974).

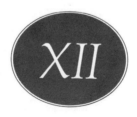

I asked Shag, "Can he hear me? His eyelashes flut-
ter . . . ," and I remembered a story we had heard in
Peking about a high official who, in the midst of pressing
state affairs, called regularly at the hospital where a comrade, a co-worker since the early days of the revolution,
had lain in a coma for weeks before her death. The doctors in charge cautioned him to save his time. "She doesn't
know you're here," they said. His reply was, "How do
you *know* she doesn't?"

"Does he *know*, Shag?" I asked.

"He may. He may not. But he's out of pain now. A coma
is an anesthetic."

"I'm glad. I hope he goes then, like this, not hurting."

He did. He never woke up. I talked to him a lot those
last three days, stroking his eyebrows, the little scar on his
temple. (I never knew where that came from and had
always meant to ask. I think he got it as a teen-ager when

he cracked up his sister Mildred's fiancé's car—and her engagement—and had to sell his saxophone as well as his summer's freedom to pay the damages.) Christopher and the Chinese were there when he died, silently in sleep, at 2:20 that bleak morning of February 15. It was Chris who woke me up.

"Mom . . . Pop died." He choked as the words came out, as I struggled into wakefulness. Then he went to tell his sister.

The Chinese were gathered in the "petit salon." I entered the bedroom alone. Afterward, after I had said good-bye (it was true, he wasn't there any more—the connections had snapped), I went out and kissed the doctors and nurses. When I did, I found each face wet with tears. I thought of Erh-wei and Little Ling; they were close by in Peking.

That night Chen Chih-fan and Wang Ching came with messages from China. We stood together while the ambassador read them aloud in Chinese and Lin Kuang-tai translated into English:

"Mrs. Lois Snow,
Please accept my deep condolences and heartfelt sympathy on the untimely passing away of Mr. Edgar Snow from illness.

Mr. Snow was a friend of the Chinese people. He exerted unremitting efforts throughout his life and made important contributions in promoting the mutual understanding and friendship between the Chinese and American peoples. His memory will live forever in the hearts of the Chinese people.

Mao Tse-tung
February 16, 1972"

"Mrs. Lois Snow,

We were shocked to learn of the untimely passing away of our respected friend Mr. Edgar Snow. At this moment of grief, Comrade Chiang Ching, Comrade Teng Ying-chao and myself extend to you our deep condolences and heartfelt sympathy.

Mr. Snow's life was a testimony to the sincere friendship between the Chinese and American peoples. Back in the period of the Chinese People's National-Democratic Revolution, he already entered into friendship with China's revolutionary forces. Breaking through the numerous obstacles of that time, he enthusiastically introduced to the American and other peoples the Chinese revolutionary struggles and the 25-thousand-li Long March of the Chinese Worker-Peasant Red Army, which were undertaken under the leadership of Chairman Mao Tse-tung. After the liberation of our country, he came again on several visits and reported the progress of the people's revolutionary cause of New China led by Chairman Mao. His writings were widely appreciated both in China and abroad. Even during his serious illness, he never ceased turning his mind to working for better understanding and friendship between the Chinese and American peoples. The Chinese people will not forget such an old friend of theirs.

Mr. Snow has left us, but we believe that the friendship between the Chinese and American peoples, for which he worked all his life, will certainly grow daily.

We hope you and your children will turn sorrow into strength and continue to work for the fulfillment of Mr. Snow's mission.

Chou En-lai
February 16, 1972"

"Mrs. Edgar Snow
1262 Eysins
Vaud, Switzerland

Just received your grievous message of the untimely

passing away of our most sincere friend who staunchly supported our struggle against native fascist reaction and Japanese military invasion during our war of resistance. Our strong friendship symbolized also mutual support in the just cause of the Chinese and American peoples. I am certain you and your children will continue to fulfill the task he has bequeathed to you, that of promoting understanding and friendship between our two great peoples. Please take comfort in the knowledge that the memory of Edgar Snow will remain forever green in the hearts of the Chinese people.

Soong Ching-ling
February 16, 1972"

I sent back my thanks, heartfelt but inadequate. Only the one who lay lifeless upstairs could have found the right words.

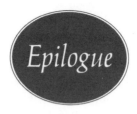

Epilogue

A few years ago Jessica Mitford presented Americans with a book full of shocking facts concerning the exploitative and degrading funeral practices in our United States.* I don't know how it is in the rest of Europe, but the Swiss "way of death" is one of dignified simplicity. That was the way we wanted it; that was the way it was done, with no complications, little expense, in privacy, with complete cooperation from the authorities in charge of the arrangements.

The Chinese dressed Ed in the light-blue "Christmas" pajamas over his favorite black *après*-ski turtleneck sweater. For three days he lay in the bed in which he had died, and those who wanted to say good-bye came up to the small room where a bowl of flowers cast a glow. Ed's sister Mildred came from Kansas City with her husband, Claude

* *The American Way of Death* (New York: Simon & Schuster, 1963; Fawcett World Library's Crest Books paperback, 1969).

136

Mackey, and Chips Snow Notman from Boston, representing her family and her father, Ed's brother Howard being prevented from travel by his wife's illness. I felt untold relief that we could be at home together, that the precious quick-passing hours were untarnished by funeral ritualism. On the fourth morning the body was placed in a plain wood box—as Ed's grandfather's must have been in Missouri years ago—and we followed the hearse, Mildred, Chips, Sian, Chris and I in the station wagon, Claude, Kashin, Shag and Joan driving behind. We took the lake road to Lausanne, patchy with memories for me as I looked out the car window: over there we had had a picnic; there a flat tire in the snow; in that house we had dined with someone long since gone away and the name forgotten; that was the spot where on the way to the airport I had made a U-turn at a speed I don't care to admit on the morning Ed, bound for China, remembered his passport was back home in another pair of pants. The lake was lilac, spring-touched. We walked around a garden for the few minutes it takes to dispose of a man's body—and then we went home.

There were four memorial services. The first, a public tribute two days before the American presidential visit, was held at the Great Hall of the People in Peking—the first time that significant building had been used in ceremonial tribute to a foreigner.

The second was in Grand Sacconex on the outskirts of Geneva. There, flowers arranged in the center of the John Knox Foyer (where Ed had spoken to its international students in times past) were a concession to ritual—we asked publicly that donations be made to La Sanitaire Centrale to recompense in whatever small way the destruction of Vietnam. Friends from around the world sat in soft shadows as Ambassador Chen read the messages from Mao Tse-tung, Chou En-lai and Soong Ching-ling. Dr. Grey Dimond spoke for those in the United States who had known and loved the man; Gilbert Etienne for Switerland, our second home; K. S. Karol and Han Suyin for Europe and the East; and Charles Harper, director of the foyer, read the words I couldn't bring myself, yet, to speak aloud. George Hatem's brief words represented two worlds.

On March 27, in the late afternoon, a similar memorial, planned by close friends, was held at the United Nations chapel in New York City. Sian had returned to school in Ohio then; Chris, Kashin and I were in Peking. We heard of the beauty of the ceremony, the spray of dogwood blossoms—Ed's favorites—like a single tree, the simple majesty of the Guarneri Quartet's music. There Ambassador Huang Hua spoke along with Edmund Clubb, Hans Maeder, Mary Heathcote, Chen Yuan-chi, Norman Rose, Tom Crane and Joan Chandler.

The fourth memorial is best described through the letter I received from Margaret Parton, a special neighbor to us in our early days of marriage and parenthood at Sneden's Landing:

> Yesterday, seventeen of us met at Sally Tompkins' house at 11:00 A.M. They were: Sally, Katy and Norman Rose and their son Jack, Jean and Hu White, Nancy Hiatt, Bill and Kitty Plageman, Jane and Lennie Schwartz, Dorothy and Harry Davis, Helen Zimbalist, Goesta and Janet Wollin. . . . After coffee we all sat around Sally's big living room and talked about the things we remembered. About Ed's making wine ("which exploded before we could drink it"); Ed and Sam Zim-

balist raiding Brooksie's refrigerator; Ed swimming in the Hudson against the tide; Ed and Sam's plans for a floating restaurant and theatre on the river. Norman remembered about how he had loaned his apartment to Ed once, and had come back two weeks after Ed had gone—and found the oven on. And Dorothy remembered how Ed had once stayed at their little house in Piermont and how when she returned she found coffee cups in odd places, like under the couch. And we all agreed that Ed could be so organized in his work, and so thorough, *because* he was absent-minded about trivia.

Goesta spoke very movingly about Ed's sense of *now*, rather than past or present. We talked of the sadness of his dying just at the time when his life's work was reaching fruition, and yet of the happiness he must have had in knowing that he had had so much to do with the rapprochement he so desired. We talked of his optimism, and Harry remembered that Ed had said, "We will have one year of progress in every one hundred." Hu White told a story of how Ed had once given him an evasive answer to a difficult question about China and the next morning had phoned to correct it, in the interest of honesty and accuracy.

We remembered sadness too, and persecution. We remembered Ed's deep love of his children and his strong desire to stay alive long enough to see them grow up. We recalled the time that Chris received a failing grade because he disagreed with a stupid teacher about China, and of how good you both were about it. We talked of Ed's warm laughter, and I retold the story about Jimmy Sheean's and Ed's stopped watches, which they took to be an occult sign and which Nehru dismissed with an easy, "You both need new watches."

I had brought *Journey to the Beginning* and Norman read a passage I liked—the long one at the very end of the book, where he speaks of his faith in the people of China, and of the need for peace in the world. That was the peak moment of the meeting. At the end Norman read the inscription on the title page, about "the end is the beginning."

Then we all said, "God bless Ed," and went home. I really do think that we felt that for an hour we had somehow re-created him in that room and that he was with us, as he always will be in our hearts.

Now when I walk into our garden alone, looking upward at sun or moon or evening star, I no longer fear my death as I did once—because Ed has gone through his—but I realize more the need to act quickly, while I live, to change as best I can the loneliness, the selfishness, that distort the potential worth of all men's lives. The feeling is not new, but it has assumed new dimensions because of what happened to us when the Chinese came. If the telling of this personal story affects others as the events affected us, it has been worth the recalling.

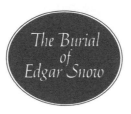

The Burial
of
Edgar Snow

On Friday, October 19, 1973, when the afternoon sun was misty in an autumn sky, a part of Edgar Snow returned forever to the campus of Peking University. As a young man he had taught in the department of journalism on these same grounds, at what was then called Yenching University. Almost forty years later a brief ceremony was conducted in the small garden where his ashes were placed beneath a white jade marble stone on which is inscribed: "In Memory of Edgar Snow, an American Friend of the Chinese People. 1905–1972." Above the English lettering the words are repeated in the Chinese calligraphy of Premier Chou En-lai, who wrote the brief text.

In his autobiography, *Journey to the Beginning,* Edgar Snow tells of the nearly two years in the '30s that he spent on this campus "in touch with modern Chinese youth and thought. Yenching was an upper-class institution," he wrote, "whose students normally should have been political conservatives. But as the national crisis deepened, and class war merged with Japan's conquests in the North, a wave of radicalism began to spread there. By 1935 Yenching had unexpectedly become the birthplace of student protests which touched off a nationwide 'rebellion of youth.' . . . Yenching had evolved from a missionary institution but was moving toward complete Chinese control, in accordance with the liberal ideals of its principal founder, Dr. J. Leighton Stuart, who was to be America's last resident ambassador at Nanking before the Communists took power. Stuart was largely responsible for raising the American funds to build Yenching and also for its distinguished architecture, a fine example of traditional Chinese, modified by Western materials and interior fittings and improvements. It was built in part on the site of the *Yuan-ming-yuan* and retained some of the original landscaping, including a lovely lake in the center of the garden-like campus. On that lake on sunny winter days we used to watch aging Manchu retainers from Hai-tien give fascinating exhibitions of figure-skating. . . ."

Yenching has since blended into the larger whole of Peking University, the Manchu retainers have given way to revolutionaries, and today the lakeside echoes with the chatter and laughter of a new generation of students, "tempered," as they say, by the struggle of the Great Proletarian Cultural Revolution.

In 1970 we had walked together, Ed and I, on the willow-lined road that circles that same lake. We paused beside a dusty-pink pavilion to gaze through its arch onto the expanse of sunlit water. Behind us, on a slight elevation reached by stones that serve as steps, lay a grassy glade framed by pines and hidden from our view. Three years have passed since that moment and the quiet spot is now a memorial to the American from Missouri who, in difficult times, had helped explain the Chinese Communist revolution to people across the seas, and to many native Chinese concerned but confused by the shaking events within their own country. The Chinese never forgot Ed's breakthrough into the blockaded Northwest to see for himself the survivors of the Long March, nor the account he gave to the world in *Red Star Over China*.

When their friend died, on February 15, 1972, the Chinese leaders offered their country as a final resting place of honor and respect. It was as simple as that. During the year I took to consider that offer, they waited, with understanding, for a reply. I discussed with the children, with Ed's family and close friends, where his ashes belonged, seeking to maintain the objectivity, the internationality of Ed's life and work.

It would have been easy and comforting to immediately accept the offer from Peking. Later I learned that many people believed I had done so when I went to China a month after Ed's death. But I had gone, with my sister and my son, solely to express our gratitude for the magnificent help the Chinese had given us in a time of sorrow and pain.

During the months of indecision I kept returning to a passage in *Journey to the Beginning*: "China had claimed a part of me even if I could make no claim on her. In place of my youthful ignorance of meanings of words and statistics there were real scenes and personalities—until famine now meant a naked young girl with breasts a million years old, and horror meant an army of rats I saw feasting on the suppurating flesh of still-living soldiers left helpless and untended on a charred battlefield; until rebellion meant the fury I felt when I saw a child turned into a pack animal and forced to walk on all fours, and 'Communism' was a youthful peasant I knew fighting to avenge the execution of 56 members of his clan-family, held jointly responsible when three of its sons joined the Red Army; until war was the slit belly of a girl ravished and thrown naked before me on the streets of Chapei, and murder was the yellow corpse of an unwanted baby tossed onto a garbage heap in an alley near the Ministry of Health; until Japan's 'anti-Communist leadership in Asia' was the feet and arms of orphan girls buried in the debris of a building bombed before my eyes, and inhumanity the laughter of idle men in silk watching one beggar choke another to death in a street fight in Szechuan over a handful of leftover rice; until I had seen dark frozen fear and cowardice in myself and courage and resolution in lowly men and women I had once childishly supposed my inferiors.

"Yes, I would be part of that. And part of me would always remain with China's tawny hills, her terraced emerald fields, her island temples seen in the early morning mist, a few of her sons and daughters who had trusted or loved me, her bankrupt cheerful civilized peasants who had sheltered and fed me, her brown, ragged, shining-eyed children, the equals and the lovers I had known, and above all the lousy, unpaid, hungry, despised, peasant foot-soldier who in the mysterious sacrifice of his own life alone now gave value to all life and put the stamp of nobility upon the struggle of a great people to survive and to go forward.

"Yes, I was proud to have known them, to have straggled across a continent with them in defeat, to have wept with them and still to share a faith with them. But I was not and could never be one of them. A man who gives himself to be the possession of an alien land . . . lives a Yahoo life . . . I was an American."

And so I hesitated to totally commit him in death where he had not been totally committed in life, for he had loved China and he had loved America and had felt the claim of each.

It was Ed who made the decision. Sometime before he became ill, long before he died, he wrote a brief note and tucked it among personal papers which he addressed to me. My sister and I came across them last summer as we were going through his files. At the end of the note he had written. "I love China. I should like part of me to stay there after death as it always did during life. America fostered and nourished me. I should like part of me placed by the Hudson River, before it enters the Atlantic to touch Europe and all the shores of mankind of which I felt a part, as I have known good men in almost every land." Part of him belonged in China, part belonged to his native land.

The Chinese not only understood this, they asked me to designate the place I thought suitable for that part of him that would rest in their country. I replied with three choices: Pao-an, the little village where Ed had first encountered Mao Tse-tung and Chou En-lai; Sian, the provincial capital of Shensi, from where Ed and George Hatem started their trip farther north in 1936—and whose name was given to our daughter, Sian; and Peking, where Ed acquired a new sense of mankind as he lived in and watched the people's struggle for freedom from foreign aggression and internal greed.

With the thought and consideration that goes into decision in China today, Peking was agreed upon as the most accessible site. The "conventional" burial place in this city is Papaoshan Cemetery—if one is a revolutionary hero or martyr. It was difficult to say no when this honor was proffered my husband, but he was neither a hero nor a martyr. He was not in a true sense a revolutionary, though his life was a "commitment against fascism, nazism and imperialism everywhere." As a writer he became teacher and educator, making "the shattering discovery that what any man writes or says can, under certain circumstances, lead people, even complete strangers, to actions which might end in speedy death. I felt [he wrote] personally answerable to the Chinese whose lives I had wittingly or unwittingly helped to place in peril. As I heard of friends and students killed in the war I realized that my own writing had taken on the nature of political action."

Participating always in the present, his eyes were constantly on the future molders of the world he would help make and leave behind. Many shadowed days were brightened by thoughtful words sent to him from youths who had responded to his books. What happened to him as a young man formed the mature battler who refused to dilute harsh truth even in the face of skepticism and scorn. I asked that he be placed somewhere at Peking University where he would be with the young. The Chinese agreed.

We gathered there that Friday, old and young and middle-aged, Chinese and foreigners—Japanese and Swedish, Canadians and English, Chileans from a country recently wrecked by military fascists and a German who long ago had left a Nazi-corrupted homeland and settled in the East, American visitors newly welcomed and American residents from the past.

In front of us, on either side of the memorial stone, traditional Chinese wreaths formed a wall of silk flowers and white ribbons; they were from Mao Tse-tung, "In tribute to Edgar Snow"; from Soong Ching-ling, Chou En-lai and Chu Teh, from Teng Ying-chao, Chiang Ching, Chiao Kuan-hua, Kuo Mo-jo, Li Fuchun, Liao Cheng-chih, from the Revolutionary Committee of Peking City, the journalists of Peking, and the students and teachers of Peking University—a wealth of friends whose paths had crisscrossed Ed's life in hard days and good, since he first set foot on China's soil. There were wreaths from family and friends far away, and beside the stone, like a burst of spring, lay a mound of fresh blossoms from "Christopher and Sian to Poppa" and from "Lois to Ed."

Liao Cheng-chih, old friend and old revolutionary, spoke for China: "Edgar Snow was an old friend of the Chinese people. For several decades, both in the years of hardship during the Chinese revolution and in the years after the founding of new China, he consistently exerted unremitting efforts and made important contributions in promoting mutual understanding and friendship between the Chinese and American peoples. His life bore testimony to the true friendship between the Chinese and American peoples. A year and more has elapsed since the death of Edgar Snow. During this peroid Sino-U.S. relations have been improved to some extent, and friendly contacts between the peoples of China and the United States have been increasing daily. We are convinced that this friendship between our two peoples, for which Edgar Snow worked all his life, will grow continuously."

My few words included my heart. "In Peking University, where he once taught the young, he now lies at rest, where other youths are benefiting from the sacrifices and struggles of past students. May those here at present and in the future—youths from many lands—use this garden as he would want it used—for rest, for play, for study, for work, in that same spirit that brought about the liberation of the country he loved."

As I spoke I could see the grave, handsome face of Chou En-lai, the sweet, strong features of Teng Ying-chao, and Sian in between, her young brow marked by her father's death. I thought of Christopher, at school in London, as my eyes passed over the solemn faces of students and teachers representing the university. In that communion of thought and acknowledgment was the essence of Edgar Snow's life in China.

In the late spring of 1974, accompanied by different friends and family, I went to Ed's beloved Hudson River and there placed that other part of him that belongs to his native land.

About the Author

Lois Wheeler Snow was born in Stockton, California. She was educated there and received her B.A. degree from the University of the Pacific. She received a scholarship to the Neighborhood Playhouse in New York City and studied there with Sanford Meisner, Herbert Berghof, Martha Graham and David Pressman. A founding member of The Actors Studio, she has appeared in many Broadway, film and television productions.

She married Edgar Snow in 1949. Their children are a son, Christopher, and a daughter, Sian ("Western Peace"). Mrs. Snow went to the People's Republic of China for the first time in 1970, with her husband, and spent five months there. She has visited that country on two other occasions. Among the publications her articles have appeared in are *Vogue, The Nation, Saturday Review, Le Monde* and *The New Republic*. Her previous book, *China On Stage*, was published in 1972.